T0344438

ULTRASOUND PHYSICS
AND TECHNOLOGY

For Elsevier

Commissioning Editor: Claire Wilson
Development Editor: Catherine Jackson
Project Manager: Jane Dingwall
Designer: Kirsteen Wright
Illustration Manager: Gillian Richards
Illustrator: David Gardner

ULTRASOUND PHYSICS AND TECHNOLOGY

TECHNOLOGY

How, Why and When

Vivien Gibbs DCR, DMU, MA, MBA
Senior Lecturer, Faculty of Health and Life Sciences,
University of the West of England, Bristol, UK

David Cole TDCR, DMU, BSc, MSc
Postgraduate Medical Ultrasound Programme Director,
Division of Radiography, Faculty of Health,
University of Central England, Birmingham, UK

Antonio Sassano BSc, MSc, AVT
Senior Lecturer, Faculty of Health and Life Sciences,
University of the West of England, Bristol, UK

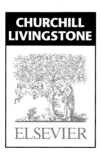

Edinburgh • London • New York • Oxford • Philadelphia • St Louis • Sydney • Toronto 2009

CHURCHILL
LIVINGSTONE
ELSEVIER

First published 2009, © Elsevier Limited. All rights reserved.

ISBN 978 0 7020 3041 3

British Library Cataloguing in Publication Data
A catalogue record for this book is available from the British Library

Library of Congress Cataloging in Publication Data
A catalog record for this book is available from the Library of Congress

Notice
Knowledge and best practice in this field are constantly changing. As new research and experience broaden our knowledge, changes in practice, treatment and drug therapy may become necessary or appropriate. Readers are advised to check the most current information provided (i) on procedures featured or (ii) by the manufacturer of each product to be administered, to verify the recommended dose or formula, the method and duration of administration, and contraindications. It is the responsibility of the practitioner, relying on their own experience and knowledge of the patient, to make diagnoses, to determine dosages and the best treatment for each individual patient, and to take all appropriate safety precautions. To the fullest extent of the law, neither the Publisher nor the Authors assumes any liability for any injury and/or damage to persons or property arising out of or related to any use of the material contained in this book.

The Publisher

ELSEVIER your source for books, journals and multimedia in the health sciences
www.elsevierhealth.com

Working together to grow libraries in developing countries
www.elsevier.com | www.bookaid.org | www.sabre.org

ELSEVIER   BOOK AID International   Sabre Foundation

The Publisher's policy is to use **paper manufactured from sustainable forests**

Printed in China

Contents

Introduction to diagnostic ultrasound

1

CONTENTS

The growth in the use of ultrasound as a diagnostic imaging tool has been rapid. Until 30 years ago ultrasound examinations were rarely performed in the hospital setting, but now this method of diagnosis is routine, and comprises over 25 per cent of diagnostic imaging examinations undertaken in the investigation of disease. A number of factors have contributed to this success, but chief among them is the relative simplicity of the process involved in obtaining diagnostic images.

A wide range of healthcare professionals now use ultrasound as a diagnostic tool. However, any practitioner using diagnostic ultrasound needs to have an understanding of the fundamental principles underlying the physical production of sound waves and echoes, in order to become fully competent in the diagnosis of information produced by the technique. This book seeks to provide the reader with the information required to underpin the practice of sonography in a format that is straightforward and easily accessible.

AUDIBLE SOUND

Sound is a form of energy which causes a mechanical disturbance in the form of vibration of molecules within a medium. In order to be transmitted, sound requires a medium containing molecules, and therefore cannot travel through a vacuum. The production of sound requires a vibrating object, such as a tuning fork, which when physically struck will vibrate. It will then cause adjacent air molecules to vibrate, and these in turn will cause their neighboring molecules to vibrate. This disturbance will spread through the air as a *longitudinal wave*. This means that the wave travels from the source of the vibration, parallel to the direction in which the particles vibrate. The phase of the wave when the molecules are pushed together is called compression, and when apart, rarefaction.

ULTRASOUND

Ultrasound is the name given to high-frequency sound waves, which are above the human hearing range. Diagnostic ultrasound travels in a similar way to audible sound. It consists of minute mechanical vibrations (pulses of ultrasound) which are transmitted into the body. As the ultrasound wave propagates (travels) through the body, it causes a local displacement of molecules within the medium. Figure 1.1 shows the changes occurring within a medium as the sound travels through it.

During its journey, the sound wave will encounter different types of tissue and, depending on the density of the tissue (how closely the molecules of the material are packed together), so the speed at which the sound travels will alter. This feature is known as the acoustic impedance of the material. The denser the medium, the greater the acoustic impedance, and the faster the sound will travel. Therefore ultrasound will travel faster in bone than in fat, for example.

The point at which the tissue type changes (the interface) is where there is a change in acoustic impedance (and a change in speed of travel of the sound), and this will cause part of the pulse to be reflected back in the form of an echo, with the remainder traveling on through the body (see Fig. 1.2). The larger the difference in acoustic impedance between two tissues, the more sound will be reflected back to the transducer and the less sound will carry on traveling through the tissue. These returning echoes are converted into a visual display and used to form a sectional image. This sequence of events is known as the pulse-echo principle.

Diagnostic ultrasound is a form of radiation because it uses energy emitted from a source.

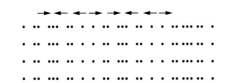

Fig. 1.1 • Areas of compression and rarefaction in a medium as the molecules are displaced

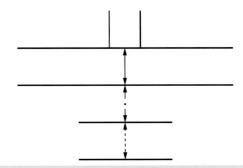

Fig. 1.2 • Echoes are returned when the sound wave encounters an interface between two tissues of differing density

However, since sound is not related to the electromagnetic spectrum, there is no tissue ionization, and the technique is therefore free from the hazards associated with X-ray imaging.

The History of Ultrasound

By the early twentieth century, the existence of inaudible high-frequency sound waves had been established, and in 1916 the first working version of a marine sonar (**so**und **na**vigation and **r**anging) system was used during the First World War to detect enemy submarines. From this, a new technique was developed for industry using high-frequency pulse-echo techniques which were applied to the detection of flaws in metallic structures.

Research progressed into using the technique for biological therapeutic and diagnostic applications, but it was not until the early 1950s that the first clinical images were published. Because air does not transmit ultrasound waves efficiently, the air interface between the transducer and the patient's skin was initially a problem. Early scanning techniques required the patient to be immersed in a bath of water in order to provide good transmission of sound waves into the body (see Fig. 1.3).

However, as this was an inconvenient technique for routine clinical use, the first contact compound B-scanner (using olive oil as a lubricant) was developed in the late 1950s (see Fig. 1.4). This equipment used a single crystal, mounted on the end of an articulating arm (see Fig 1.5), to produce static images. Each scan was time consuming to complete, as it required the operator to move the crystal across the area of interest in a linear sweep, in order to provide sufficient cross-sectional information to make a diagnosis.

Early ultrasound equipment visual displays used storage oscilloscopes which produced bi-stable (black and white) images (see Fig. 1.6). It was only in the 1970s that gray scale imaging was introduced, enabling the display of a wide range of echo amplitudes. More subtle variations in tissue density were provided by these images, enabling the diagnosis of a wider range of disease processes.

Real-time scanning systems were introduced in the mid 1970s, which not only enabled the visualization of moving structures, but also helped to speed up the examination time. Dynamic sonographic information was available for the first time, greatly enhancing the use of ultrasound as a diagnostic tool.

During these developments, research into the application of Doppler techniques was ongoing for many years, and the technique began to be used routinely for the detection and measurement of blood flow during the 1980s. Ongoing research into this, together with the use of micro-bubbles as a contrast medium, continues to expand the diagnostic applications of sonography.

Safety of Ultrasound

The ultrasound beam is potentially hazardous to the patient. As it travels through the body the beam interacts with tissue, and if exposure is

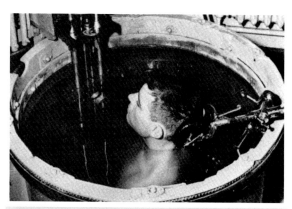

Fig. 1.3 • A patient being scanned in a waterbath in 1954 (Reproduced from Shirley et al 1978.)

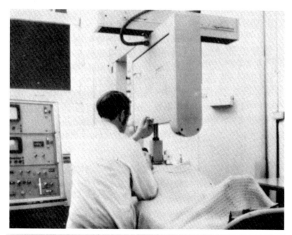

Fig. 1.4 • A contact compound B-scanning machine (Reproduced from Shirley et al 1978.)

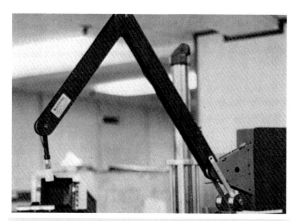

Fig. 1.5 • A single crystal transducer mounted on an articulating arm (Reproduced from Shirley et al 1978.)

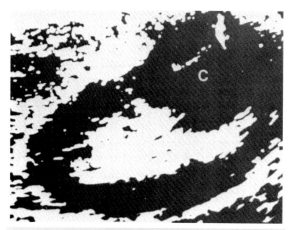

Fig. 1.6 • A bi-stable image of a renal cyst (Reproduced from Shirley et al 1978.)

3

sustained and of sufficient intensity, it has the potential to cause a lasting biological effect. The implications of many of the processes that occur are not yet fully understood, however two of the effects that have been observed are caused by thermal and mechanical processes. The thermal effects arise because some of the ultrasound energy is converted into heat, causing an increase in tissue temperature. The mechanical processes are a result of the presence of air in soft tissues (such as the lungs or intestines) which can cause damage to cells as the air bubbles expand under the influence of the ultrasound beam (see Chapter 12 on Ultrasound safety).

The degree of damage caused by these effects depends on a number of factors, including the length of the scan, the type of tissue being scanned and the power of the ultrasound beam. Anyone performing an ultrasound scan therefore needs to be aware of the possible hazards involved, in order to take the necessary precautions to limit possible damage to the patient.

Ultrasound Equipment

The device which transmits the sound into the patient and detects the returning echoes is called the transducer. The term transducer means a device that converts one form of energy into another. The primary component of the transducer is the piezoelectric crystal which enables the conversion of electrical pulses into mechanical energy (sound), and will also convert mechanical energy into electrical signals. Most ultrasound equipment now uses pulsed sound, which means that a voltage is applied to the crystal for a fraction of a second. This distorts the crystal and a pulse of ultrasound is therefore produced. The crystal will then relax while it is waiting to receive a returning echo. Only 1 per cent of the operating time is spent by the transducer transmitting sound, whereas 99 per cent of the time is spent listening for echoes.

Echoes detected by the transducer give rise to very small voltage signals in the piezoelectric crystal. By measuring the time it takes for an echo to arrive back at the transducer, the depth of the echo can be calculated by the equipment. These signals are then amplified, converted into a digital format and stored as digital numbers in a computer memory known as a scan converter. Each digital number will be assigned to an individual pixel according to how large the returning echo is, and the digital number for each pixel determines the shade of gray used to represent it on the display. Considerable processing and manipulation of this echo data has to occur before it can be meaningfully displayed. Processing takes place either before storage (pre-processing) or after (post-processing). Many processing functions can be manipulated by the operator (see Chapter 10 on Instrumentation and controls) and have a considerable effect on the quality of the image. Incorrect use of these controls can lead to the production of artifacts and misinterpretation of the image (see Chapter 9 on Artifacts).

The Image

After the returning echo signals have been electronically processed and amplified they are displayed as shades of gray, ranging from black to white. Most systems have the capability to display up to 64 shades of gray on a monitor. Stronger reflectors will be displayed as white on an image, weaker echoes will be less bright, and areas with no echoes will be portrayed as black.

All ultrasound images are composed of many lines of echo data, placed closely together so that the image appears continuous. The area of the patient displayed on any image is limited by the section through which the beam will sweep. The width is determined by the type of the transducer, and the depth by the length of time for which the echoes are recorded following transmission of a pulse. The depth is variable according to operator requirements, but usually has a maximum of 25 cm.

The plane that an ultrasound image represents is the section through which the ultrasound beam sweeps, and this is determined by the position and orientation of the transducer. During scanning, the operator is required to move the transducer in order to view images in at least two planes, and to use this information to build up a mental three-dimensional image of the area being surveyed.

In order to understand the basic principles of diagnostic ultrasound it is important to have a working knowledge of the basic physics of sound, and the way in which high-frequency sound interacts with biological tissue. The following chapters will explore in more detail some of these principles.

Reference

Shirley I, Blackwell R, Cusick G et al 1978 A user's guide to diagnostic ultrasound. Pitman Medical, London.

Further reading

Brown TG 1960 Direct contact ultrasonic scanning techniques for the visualisation of abdominal masses. In: Proceedings of the 2nd International Conference on Medical Electronics. Illiffe & Sons Ltd, London, p 358.

Howry DH, Bliss WR 1952 Ultrasonic visualisation of soft tissue structures of the body. Journal of Laboratory and Clinical Medicine 40:579.

Meire HB, Farrant P 1982 Basic clinical ultrasound. BIR Teaching Series No 4.

Principles and physics of ultrasound imaging–
simple terminology definitions

Absorption: This is the major cause of attenuation. Absorption occurs when ultrasound energy is lost to tissues by its conversion to heat. Higher frequency waves undergo greater absorption.

Acoustic impedance: A property of all substances and is equal to the product of the tissue density and the speed of sound. Comparatively speaking, two substances with greater differences in acoustic impedance produce stronger 'echoes' or reflected waves than two similar substances. Structures of different acoustic impedance (for example, gallbladder and gallstone) are easier to distinguish from one another than two structures of similar acoustic impedance (for example, liver and kidney).

Acoustic power: The rate of flow of energy through the cross-sectional area of the beam.

Acoustic waves: These are the vibrations that occur as a result of the rapid forward and reverse vibrations of the transducer, and which result in a number of longitudinal waves being transmitted. The transducer causes molecules in the medium through which it is passing to vibrate in a series of rhythmic, mechanical compressions (high-pressure regions) and rarefactions (low-pressure regions). These vibrations are commonly known as acoustic waves.

Acoustic window: An area of the patient that enhances ultrasound transmission and provides optimal scanning access to the area of interest. To improve image quality, ultrasound transmission should be as uniform as possible and areas which are likely to cause artifacts (such as ribs or bowel gas) should be avoided.

ALARA: An acronym for 'as low as reasonably achievable', referring to the principle of keeping power and exposure time to a minimum while acquiring the necessary clinical information.

Amplitude: The height of a wave. The amplitude and intensity of sound represent the energy associated with the sound wave. The greater the amplitude or intensity, the more the energy, and the 'louder' the sound. Increasing the acoustic power will increase both the intensity and the amplitude (see Fig. 2.1).

Anechoic: Areas on the image showing no internal echoes, appearing dark or black on the image.

Artifacts: In the context of ultrasound, artifacts are echo signals whose displayed position on the image does not correspond to the actual position of a reflector in the body, or whose displayed brightness is not indicative of the reflecting or scattering properties of the region from which the echo originated. Artifacts are a result of the following programmed machine assumptions:

1 The speed of sound propagation is the same in all tissue types
2 The ultrasound beam travels in straight lines
3 The time taken after emission of a pulse for an echo to return to the transducer

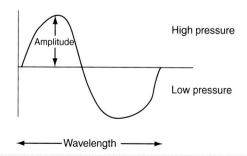

Fig. 2.1 · Sound can be depicted as a sine wave

from an interface is directly related to the distance of the interface from the transducer

4 Attenuation of sound in tissue is uniform
5 All echoes detected by the transducer have arisen from the central axis of the beam
6 An echo generated at an interface returns directly in a straight line to the transducer without generating any secondary echoes
7 The intensity or strength of the returning echo is proportional to the density of the reflector generating the echo.

Attenuation: The process that occurs as a sound wave travels through a medium; it loses energy, and as a result, its intensity and amplitude decrease, and it becomes attenuated. Attenuation is proportional to the frequency of the sound wave and the distance that the wave travels. The higher the frequency and the further the wave travels, the greater the attenuation. Attenuation results from three main effects: absorption, reflection, and scattering.

Axial resolution: This refers to reflectors that lie *along the axis* of the ultrasound beam. This resolution is dependent upon the pulse length, which is equal to the product of the number of cycles in a pulse and the wavelength. If two reflectors *along the axis* of the ultrasound beam are separated by a distance longer than half the pulse length, they will appear as two separate reflectors. If the distance between the reflectors is less than the pulse length, they will appear as one reflector. Since the wavelength and frequency are inversely related, axial resolution is improved by increasing the frequency of the transducer. Thus, high-frequency transducers have better axial resolution.

Beam former: Provides pulse delay sequences to individual elements (an element consists of a piezoelectric crystal *and* its electrical connection) to achieve focusing of the ultrasound beam.

Cavitation: The pressure oscillations produced by sound can create gas bubbles from the air dissolved in tissue fluids. If the oscillations are rapid and intense, they can cause the bubbles to expand, contract, or collapse. The potential for cavitation is related to the acoustic pressure amplitudes produced by the ultrasound system. These amplitudes are reported by the manufacturer in the operator's manual. Some scanning machines provide continuous assessment of the potential risk of bioeffects due to cavitation, by calculating the mechanical index (MI) for a given transducer in a particular mode during a scan. The MI is inversely proportional to the square root of the frequency; thus, as frequency increases, MI decreases.

Contact coupling: This can be either gel or liquid. Adequate coupling agent is needed to ensure that there is no air between the transducer and the skin.

Coronal plane: Divides the body into anterior and posterior sections, perpendicular to the sagittal.

Depth: The depth range or depth control varies the depth of the patient which is displayed on the image. The optimal depth is dependent upon beam penetration, which is determined by the transducer frequency.

Diffuse reflectors: These are also known as scatterers, and reflect sound in all directions. The brightness is not dependent on the angle of the incident beam.

Doppler shift: This is the phenomenon that occurs when sound is reflected from a moving object and the frequency of the reflected sound changes. The change in frequency is known as the Doppler shift, named after Christian Doppler, the Austrian physicist, who described it in 1842. Analysis of the Doppler shift can be used to determine the speed and direction of blood as it courses through the cardiovascular system. A *positive* Doppler shift means that the *received* frequency *exceeds* the *transmitted* frequency and that red blood cells are approaching the transducer. A *negative* Doppler shift means that the *received* frequency is *less* than the *transmitted* frequency and that the red blood cells are moving away from the transducer.

Dynamic range: This allows the range of echoes or shades of gray displayed on the screen to be decreased. This will remove low-level echoes from the display and result in an image with more contrast.

Echo: A sound wave that is reflected from a tissue interface at 90° and is received by the ultrasound transducer.

Echogenic: This is an ambiguous term and should be avoided, unless used as a comparative descriptor, e.g. increased echogenicity (meaning increased reflectivity).

Electrical shock: A damaged transducer housing, or a break in the insulation of the transducer cable, can result in a significant electrical shock to the ultrasonographer or to the patient. This bioeffect is easily prevented by regular equipment maintenance and frequent checks of the cable, transducer, and electrical connections.

Focus: To improve the resolution at a given depth, the transducer must be focused in order to narrow the beam width. This can be performed electronically by varying the number of transmitting and receiving elements and by delaying the signal once it is received from some of the elements.

Frequency: The number of cycles of acoustic waves per second. The unit of frequency is the hertz (Hz). One cycle per second is equal to 1 Hz; 10^6 cycles/second is equal to 1 megahertz (MHz). Audible sound has a frequency between 20 and 20 000 Hz, whereas ultrasound has a frequency greater than 20 000 Hz. Diagnostic ultrasound has a frequency of 2–20 MHz.

Gain: The degree of amplification of the returning echo is called the gain. Echo or signal amplification is necessary because the returning echoes are too weak to be displayed and visualized. Echoes can be strengthened by increasing the intensity of the transmitted signal (that is, increasing the power) or by increasing the amplification of the returning signal (that is, increasing the gain). Mathematically, the gain is the ratio of the signal amplitude input into the amplifier to the signal amplitude output from the amplifier. Gain is commonly expressed in decibels (dB). If the gain is increased too much, then inherent noise within the system will also be amplified, leading to poor image quality.

Heat: Absorption represents the conversion of ultrasound energy to heat. Heating is one of the mechanisms for the production of biological effects by ultrasound and is proportional to the power applied to the beam or pulse and the duration of exposure. Imaging modes using more frequent pulses (higher pulse repetition frequency (PRF)) deliver more energy or power to the patient. A number of criteria are used to indicate the amount of power or acoustical output of scanners. These criteria are specific to the system and to the manufacturer and can be found in the operator's manual. Some equipment provides continuous assessment of the potential risk of bioeffects due to heating, by calculating the thermal index (TI) for a given transducer in a particular mode during a scan. To reduce bioeffects, the TI and exposure time should be minimized. Obviously, the higher the TI, the lower the exposure time should be.

Hyperechoic: Areas on the image with more reflected echoes (brighter) than surrounding tissue.

Hypoechoic: Areas on the image with fewer reflected echoes (darker) than surrounding tissue.

Image characteristics: Image characteristics are determined by 'reflectors' and 'scatterers' of the ultrasound beam. The degree to which an area reflects, transmits, and scatters the ultrasound beam determines how brightly it is portrayed on the image.

Impedance matching layers: These layers are interfaced between the crystals and the patient to reduce the acoustical impedance mismatch between the patient and the transducer. A high acoustical impedance mismatch between the patient and transducer would create a strong reverberation artifact.

Intensity: Defined as the power per unit area and expressed in milliwatts per square centimeter.

Isoechoic: Areas on the image showing a level of reflected echoes similar to that of surrounding tissue.

Lateral resolution: This refers to reflectors that lie *perpendicular to the axis* of the ultrasound beam. The resolution is related to the beam width; that is, the wider the beam, the poorer the lateral resolution. An ultrasound beam is narrowest at its focal length, and this is where the lateral resolution will be optimum.

Overall gain control: This simple gain control increases amplification of echoes from *all depths*; it has an effect similar to increasing the power.

9

Piezoelectric effect: An effect exhibited by certain crystals with piezoelectric properties. The crystal changes shape and vibrates when a voltage is applied to it. These are the primary components of ultrasound transducers. The most common type of piezoelectric material found in ultrasound transducers is **lead zirconate titanate (PZT)**. These specialized crystals enable the transducer to convert electrical energy into acoustic energy during transmission, and to reverse the process (that is, convert acoustical energy into electrical energy) during reception. If piezoelectric materials are heated, they become depolarized and lose their piezoelectric properties. Therefore, ultrasound transducers *should not be heat sterilized*! In addition they are sensitive to mechanical shock and *should not be dropped*!

Power: Increasing the output power to the transducer produces high-intensity ultrasound pulses. This increases the amplitude of the electrical signal applied to the transducer, which has the effect of making returning echo signals from all reflectors appear brighter. The disadvantage of increasing the power is that acoustic exposure of the patient increases.

Presets: After a transducer and a type of scan (that is, abdominal, vascular, obstetric, etc.) are selected, the system can be programmed to automatically select certain controls, such as the power or gain controls. This can save time setting up the equipment for each individual patient; however, there are often occasions when the preset is not adequate and the operator therefore needs to have an understanding of the controls in order to optimize the image quality.

Propagation speed: The speed at which sound moves through a medium, and is equal to the product of wavelength and frequency. Generally, the speed depends on tissue density and is lowest in gases, higher in liquids, and highest in solids. The average speed of sound in soft tissue is 1540 m/s.

Pulse-echo principle: This refers to the process which occurs when ultrasound waves encounter an interface between two tissues with different acoustic impedances. Most of the waves are transmitted into the tissue, and part of the beam will be reflected back to the transducer. The electrical signal that is generated from those waves is proportional to the strength of the returning wave. The strength of the returning wave is proportional to the amount of difference in acoustic impedance between the two tissues at the interface. The ultrasound image is formed only by those waves that are reflected back and received by the transducer.

Pulse repetition frequency (PRF): The PRF controls the rate at which pulses of sound waves are produced and transmitted.

Pulse transmitter: Provides electrical signals to excite the piezoelectric crystals. The pulsing signals are applied at a rate known as the **pulse repetition frequency (PRF)**. The PRF varies from 500–12 000/s with the operating mode and other settings on the machine. For example, real-time gray scale imaging requires a PRF of 2000–4000/s, whereas pulsed Doppler requires a PRF of 4000–12 000/s.

Reflection: This occurs when two large structures of significantly different acoustic impedance (such as an organ boundary) form an interface, the interface becomes a reflector, and some of the wave energy is reflected back to the transducer. The energy remaining in the wave (not reflected, but transmitted beyond the interface) is decreased. Reflection occurs when a sound wave strikes an object that is larger than the wavelength.

Refraction: When the beam encounters an interface between two different tissues at an oblique angle, the beam will be deviated as it travels on through the tissue. This is known as refraction. If the angle of incidence is 90°, no refraction will occur.

Resolution: The ability of an ultrasound system to distinguish two closely spaced reflectors as separate structures is known as resolution.

Sagittal (longitudinal) plane: Divides the body into right and left sections, parallel to the long axis.

Scattering: This occurs when an ultrasound wave strikes a boundary or interface between two small structures, and the wave is scattered in different directions. Scattering occurs when a sound wave strikes an object that is equal to or smaller than the wavelength. Scattering is therefore directly related to the frequency of the wave.

Sound: Energy transmitted as a mechanical, longitudinal wave that requires a medium through which to travel (see Fig. 2.1).

Spatial resolution: The minimum distance between two adjacent features that can be detected by the imaging system.

Specular reflectors: These are strong reflectors and, as a result, the brightness of the echoes in the image is dependent on the angle of the incident beam and the reflector surface.

Temporal resolution: The ability to accurately portray movement occurring within the field of view during real-time imaging.

Texture: In B-mode scanning, the amplitudes of the returning signals are displayed on a gray scale from white (strong echo) to black (no echo perceived) and in-between shades of gray. The arrangement of reflected echoes as 'dots' on the image is referred to as the texture.

Time gain compensation (TGC) or depth gain compensation (DGC): This is required in order to compensate for the fact that signals returning from deeper reflectors will be weaker than signals returning from more shallow reflectors, because of attenuation. Increasing TGC amplifies signals more from deeper structures (that is, those that are relatively more delayed – hence, *time gain*) than it does from shallow structures (that is, less delayed).

Transaxial (transverse) plane: Divides the body into superior and inferior sections, perpendicular to the long axis.

Transducer: A device which converts one form of energy to another. An ultrasound transducer converts electrical energy into sound energy, and vice versa. It contains the piezoelectric crystals which transmit the ultrasound beam and receive the reflected echoes.

Transducer backing material: This material is placed behind the crystals to dampen vibrations from them and shorten the pulse duration.

Transducer housing: This housing consists of durable metal and plastic, enclosing the transducer to protect it from damage.

Transducer orientation: Convention dictates the orientation of the transducer relative to the patient. This results in a display which demonstrates the patient's head to the left of the screen during a sagittal (or longitudinal) scan, and the patient's right side on the left of the screen during a transaxial (or transverse) scan. Therefore images are always viewed as if from the patient's right side during a sagittal scan, and as if from the patient's feet during a transaxial scan. Transducers have an embedded indicator that must be correctly aligned with the corresponding indicator on the monitor, in order to ensure correct display of the scanning plane.

Ultrasound beam: This is composed of a **near zone** or **Fresnel zone** where the beam is cylindrical in shape (the area between the transducer and the focus); a **focal zone** (the area where the diameter of the sound beam is at a minimum and the image quality is best); and a **far zone** or **Fraunhofer zone** where the beam diverges (the area extending beyond the focus).

Wavelength: The length of one cycle, usually measured in mm. As the frequency becomes higher, the wavelength becomes shorter. Conversely, as the frequency becomes lower, the wavelength becomes longer (see Fig. 2.1).

Further reading

Hedrick WR, Hykes L, Starchman DE 1995 Ultrasound physics and instrumentation, 3rd edn. Mosby, St Louis.

Sanders RC 1991 Clinical sonography: a practical guide, 2nd edn. Little, Brown, Boston.

Zagzebski JA 1996 Essentials of ultrasound physics. Mosby-Year Book, St Louis.

The piezoelectric effect

CONTENTS

LEARNING OBJECTIVES

1 Explain what is meant by the piezoelectric effect.

2 Describe how piezoelectric crystals are used for the production and detection of sound.

3 Explain what is meant by the resonant frequency of a piezoelectric crystal.

4 Describe the factors which determine the output frequency of a piezoelectric crystal.

THE PIEZOELECTRIC EFFECT

This is the ability of a material to generate an electrical charge in response to applied pressure. When a piece of piezoelectric material is compressed a potential difference is generated across opposite faces – the one side becomes positive, the other negative (Fig. 3.1). Conversely, if an electric field is applied across the crystal it changes its shape (Fig. 3.2).

PIEZOELECTRIC MATERIALS

This property is exhibited by certain crystalline materials such as quartz, which is a naturally occurring crystal, and lead zirconate titanate, which is a man-made ceramic.

Piezoelectric materials are crystalline materials composed of dipolar molecules, which are positive at one end and negative at the other (Fig. 3.3). Normally these dipolar molecules have a random arrangement within the material and they are unable to align themselves with an applied electric field (Fig. 3.4). However, if the material is heated above the Curie temperature in the presence of an electric field, the molecules will

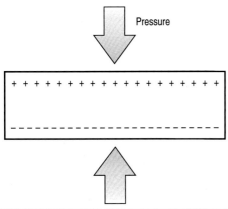

Fig. 3.1 • Compression of a piezoelectric crystal results in a potential difference across opposite faces

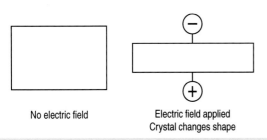

No electric field   Electric field applied
                           Crystal changes shape

Fig. 3.2 • When an electric field is applied to a piezoelectric crystal it changes its shape

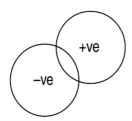

Fig. 3.3 • A dipolar molecule having positive and negative regions

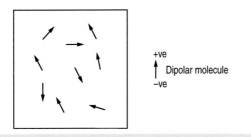

Fig. 3.4 • Random arrangement of dipolar molecules within the piezoelectric material

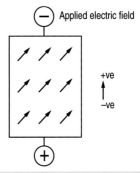

Fig. 3.5 • When material is heated above the Curie temperature in the presence of an electric field, the molecules will align themselves with the field

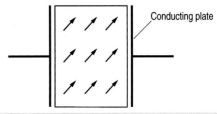

Fig. 3.6 • Opposite faces of the crystal have conducting plates attached to their surfaces. These surfaces are at right angles to the previously applied electric field

align themselves with that field. If the material is then allowed to cool below the Curie temperature, while the electric field is maintained, the molecules will remain aligned to the electric field and maintain this position even after the field is removed (see Fig. 3.5). This piezoelectric crystal can now be used in an ultrasound transducer to transmit and to detect sound. Opposite faces of the crystal have conducting plates attached to their surfaces. These surfaces are at right angles to the previously applied electric field (Fig. 3.6).

THE PIEZOELECTRIC CRYSTAL AS A TRANSMITTER OF SOUND

In this case the crystal is converting electrical energy into mechanical energy. A voltage is applied to the conducting plates causing the molecules to twist in the direction of the electric field and this causes the crystal to become thicker (Fig. 3.7). If this voltage is reversed the molecules will twist back in the opposite direction making the crystal thinner (Fig. 3.8). Applying an alternating voltage

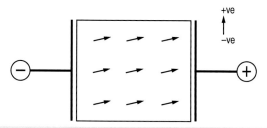

Fig. 3.7 • A voltage is applied to the conducting plates causing the molecules to twist in the direction of the electric field and this causes the crystal to become thicker

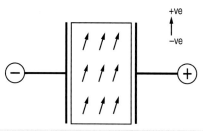

Fig. 3.8 • If this voltage is reversed the molecules will twist back in the opposite direction making the crystal thinner

to the crystal will cause it to expand and contract (oscillate) at the same frequency as the voltage, producing a continuous sound wave of that frequency. The degree of expansion and contraction is known as the amplitude of oscillation and is dependent partly on the voltage. Increasing the applied voltage increases the amplitude of oscillation. The amplitude of oscillation is also dependent on the resonant frequency of the crystal (see below).

THE PIEZOELECTRIC CRYSTAL AS A RECEIVER OF SOUND

In this case the crystal is converting mechanical energy into electrical energy. When a sound wave makes contact with a piezoelectric crystal the regions of high pressure and low pressure cause the crystal to contract and expand. This twists the dipolar molecules which results in the conducting plates becoming charged either positive and negative or negative and positive (Fig. 3.9). In other words, small voltage signals are produced from the sound wave. The size of the voltage signal

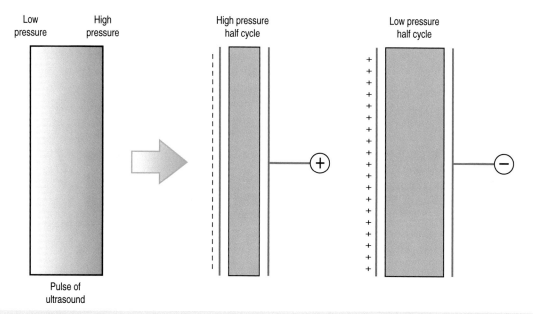

Fig. 3.9 • When a sound wave makes contact with a piezoelectric crystal it results in the conducting plates becoming charged either negative and positive or positive and negative

15

produced depends upon the amplitude (loudness or strength) of the sound wave. Sound with higher amplitude results in a signal with a higher voltage.

PRODUCTION OF A PULSED SOUND WAVE

The process described above is for the production and detection of a continuous sound wave, the frequency of the sound wave being equal to the frequency of the applied voltage. However, when producing a pulsed sound wave the crystal is subjected to a very short pulse of high voltage electricity, typically 500 V and 1 microsecond, which produces a pulse of sound approximately 2 wavelengths long. The frequency of the sound produced depends upon the thickness of the crystal. In fact, the natural frequency of the crystal is such that the wavelength of the pulse of sound emitted equals twice the thickness of the crystal.

RESONANCE

This is is the tendency of an object to oscillate at maximum amplitude at a certain frequency. For example, if a series of voltages of different frequencies are applied to a piezoelectric crystal, the surfaces of the crystal will oscillate at the frequency of the applied voltage. However, at a certain frequency the amplitude of the oscillation will be much greater than at any other frequency. This is known as the resonant frequency or natural frequency of the crystal.

FACTORS AFFECTING WAVELENGTH/ FREQUENCY

The frequency output from a piezoelectric crystal depends upon the thickness of the crystal and the type of voltage applied to the crystal. For B-mode ultrasound a short pulse of high voltage electricity is applied. This is typically 500 volts and 2 wavelengths long. In this case the crystal emits a range of frequencies, with the center frequency equal to the resonant frequency. With continuous Doppler ultrasound a continuous alternating voltage is applied to the crystal, which emits a sound wave

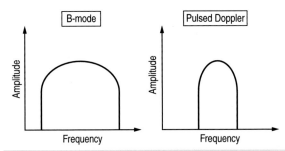

Fig. 3.10 • Amplitude versus frequency graphs for a B-mode and pulsed Doppler ultrasound

of a single frequency equal to the frequency of the applied voltage. For pulsed Doppler ultrasound a longer pulse of ultrasound is applied, typically 8–10 wavelengths long. This emits a short pulse of sound with a center frequency equal to that of the applied voltage. Although there are a range of frequencies present in this pulse, the range is narrower than that produced in B-mode imaging (Fig. 3.10).

IMPORTANT PROPERTIES OF PIEZOELECTRIC MATERIALS

Acoustic Impedance

The acoustic impedance of the piezoelectric crystal should be chosen so that it is as close to the acoustic impedance of the patient's skin as practicable. This is to ensure that there is efficient transfer of sound energy between the crystal and the patient. If there is a large acoustic impedance mismatch between crystal and the patient's skin then a large amount of energy is reflected at the interface and only a small amount transmitted. This affects both the transmission and reception of sound.

Energy Conversion Efficiency

This is the efficiency of the piezoelectric crystal to convert electrical energy into sound energy and to convert sound energy into electrical energy. Both types of conversion efficiency (electricity into sound and sound into electricity) are important in ensuring efficient production of ultrasound and sensitivity in detecting weak echoes.

SUMMARY

- The piezoelectric effect is the ability of a material to generate an electrical charge in response to applied pressure
- Piezoelectric materials also respond to an applied electric field by changes to their shape
- Piezoelectric crystals are used in the production of ultrasound by converting electrical energy into mechanical energy (sound)
- Piezoelectric crystals are used in the detection of ultrasound by converting mechanical energy (sound) into electrical energy
- Piezoelectric crystals have a natural frequency (resonant frequency) at which they produce oscillations of maximum amplitude. The resonant frequency depends upon the thickness of the crystal
- The frequency of the emitted sound depends upon the frequency of the applied voltage, the thickness of the crystal, and the type of imaging modality being used
- The ability of the crystal to produce ultrasound efficiently, transmit it into the patient, and be sensitive to weak echoes depends on the acoustic impedance of the piezoelectric crystal and its energy conversion efficiency

Acoustic impedance

4

LEARNING OBJECTIVES

1 Describe what is meant by the term acoustic impedance.

2 Explain the properties of a substance which determine its acoustic impedance.

3 List a set of body tissues in order of their acoustic impedance.

4 Describe how the amount of ultrasound energy reflected at the interface between two substances is determined by their acoustic impedances.

5 Give the meaning of the term *intensity reflection coefficient*.

6 Explain why ultrasound is good at imaging different soft tissues but poor at imaging soft tissue/bone and soft tissue/air.

Acoustic impedance (Z) is the property of a substance, which describes how the particles of that substance behave when subjected to a pressure wave, i.e. a sound wave. Acoustic impedance gives the relationship between **excess pressure** P and **particle velocity** U_0 as shown in Figure 4.1.

If the substance has densely packed particles, for example bone, then it will take a high excess pressure for them to move at a given velocity. Therefore this type of substance will have high acoustic impedance.

On the other hand if the substance has loosely packed particles, for example air, then it will take a much lower excess pressure for them to move at the same velocity. Therefore this type of substance will have low acoustic impedance.

Acoustic impedance gives a measure of the resistance a substance has to the propagation of a

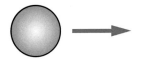

Particle p
traveling at velocity U_0

Due to excess pressure P

Fig. 4.1 • A particle subjected to excess pressure P traveling at velocity U_0. This gives the acoustic impedance formula:

$$\text{Acoustic impedance } Z = \frac{\text{EXCESS PRESSURE}}{\text{PARTICLE VELOCITY}} = \frac{P}{U_0}$$

sound wave through it. It is normally calculated from density ρ and speed of sound c as follows:

$$Z = \rho c$$

density ρ	kg/m^3
speed of sound c	m/s
acoustic impedance Z	rayls ($= kg/m^2/s$)

In this book, speed and velocity have the same meaning. The acoustic impedance of various substances is given in Table 4.1.

SUBSTANCE	ACOUSTIC IMPEDANCE IN MEGARAYLS $(kg/m^2/s) \times 10^6$	SPEED (m/s)
Air	0.0004	330
Fat	1.38	1450
Water	1.48	1480
Blood	1.61	1570
Kidney	1.62	1560
Liver	1.65	1550
Muscle	1.70	1580
Soft tissue (average)	1.63	1540
Bone	7.80	3500
PZT (Crystal)	30	3870

Note: the acoustic impedances of air and bone are very different.

Table 4.1 The acoustic impedance of various substances

ACOUSTIC IMPEDANCE AND REFLECTION

When an ultrasound beam strikes an interface between substances it is the acoustic impedances of the two substances that determine whether reflection takes place and the amount of energy reflected. The examples below illustrate this.

In substances with the same acoustic impedance there is total transmission of energy and therefore no reflection, see Figure 4.2.

In substances with a small difference in acoustic impedance a small amount of energy is reflected but the majority is transmitted, see Figure 4.3.

In substances with a large difference in acoustic impedance there is a large amount of reflected energy and a small amount of transmitted energy, see Figure 4.4.

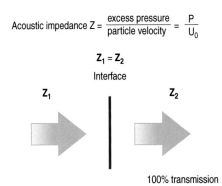

$$\text{Acoustic impedance } Z = \frac{\text{excess pressure}}{\text{particle velocity}} = \frac{P}{U_0}$$

$$Z_1 = Z_2$$

Interface

Z_1 Z_2

100% transmission

Fig. 4.2 • Total transmission of ultrasound energy as it passes across an interface between two substances of the same acoustic impedance

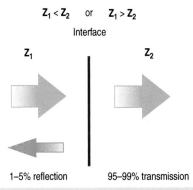

$$Z_1 < Z_2 \quad \text{or} \quad Z_1 > Z_2$$

Interface

Z_1 Z_2

1–5% reflection   95–99% transmission

Fig. 4.3 • A small amount of reflected energy and a large amount of transmitted energy as ultrasound passes across an interface between two substances with a small difference in acoustic impedance

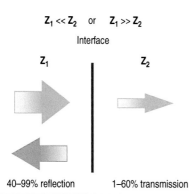

$$Z_1 \ll Z_2 \quad \text{or} \quad Z_1 \gg Z_2$$

Interface

Z_1 Z_2

40–99% reflection   1–60% transmission

Fig. 4.4 • A large amount of reflected energy and a small amount of transmitted energy as ultrasound passes across an interface between two substances with a large difference in acoustic impedance

INTENSITY REFLECTION COEFFICIENT

This gives the proportion of energy reflected from an interface between two substances and has a value between 0 and 1, where 0 = total transmission and 1 = total reflection.

The intensity reflection coefficient for various interfaces is given in Table 4.2.

For most soft tissue/soft-tissue interfaces the percentage of energy reflected is 1% or less.

THE INTENSITY REFLECTION EQUATION

This equation allows you to calculate the intensity reflection coefficient (R) for an interface between two substances providing you know their acoustic impedances.

INTERFACE	INTENSITY REFLECTION COEFFICIENT R	PERCENTAGE OF ENERGY REFLECTED (%R)
Fat/Muscle	0.0108	1.08
Bone/Muscle	0.412	41.2
Air/Soft tissue	0.999	99.9

Note the high reflection coefficients for bone/muscle and air/soft tissue.

Table 4.2 The intensity reflection coefficient for various interfaces

$$R = \frac{I_r}{I_i} = \frac{(Z_1 - Z_2)^2}{(Z_1 + Z_2)^2}$$

I_r = reflected intensity

I_i = transmitted intensity

Z_1 and Z_2 = acoustic impedances of the two substances

Example

What is the intensity reflection coefficient R for an interface between liver (Z_1 = 1.65 Mrayls) and fat (Z_2 = 1.35 Mrayls)?

$$R = \frac{(Z_1 - Z_2)^2}{(Z_1 + Z_2)^2} = \frac{(1.65 - 1.35)^2}{(1.65 + 1.35)^2} = \frac{(0.3)^2}{(3.0)^2}$$

$$= \left(\frac{0.3}{3.0}\right)^2$$

$$= (0.1)^2 = 0.01 = 1.0\%$$

ACOUSTIC IMPEDANCE AND ULTRASOUND IMAGING

The difference in acoustic impedance between two substances is known as the acoustic impedance mismatch. It is this acoustic impedance mismatch at an interface which is responsible for ultrasound energy being reflected back toward the probe and being used to produce an image.

If there is a large acoustic mismatch, e.g. between bone and muscle or air and soft tissue, then a large proportion of energy is reflected. This results in a strong echo, which produces a bright image on the display. However, very little energy is transmitted across the interface and any echoes produced beyond the interface do not have enough energy to produce an image, see Figure 4.5.

If the acoustic impedance mismatch is small, e.g. between two soft tissues, then a small proportion of energy (1% or less) is reflected. The rest of the energy is transmitted across the interface to produce further echoes from other interfaces deeper within the subject, see Figure 4.6.

From the above it can be seen that where there is a large acoustic impedance mismatch across an interface, ultrasound will not produce a useful image beyond that interface. Therefore it is not practical to use ultrasound to produce images of

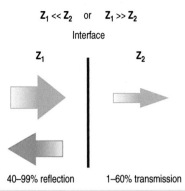

$Z_1 \ll Z_2$ or $Z_1 \gg Z_2$

Interface

Z_1 Z_2

40–99% reflection   1–60% transmission

Fig. 4.5 • Diagram showing an interface with strong reflection but poor transmission/penetration

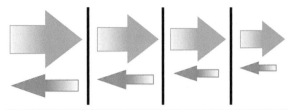

Fig. 4.6 • Diagram showing echoes reflected from a series of soft tissue/soft-tissue interfaces

soft-tissue subjects which contain gas or bone. However, ultrasound imaging is very good at discriminating between substances with small differences in acoustic impedance and is therefore excellent at differentiating between different types of soft tissues.

SUMMARY

- Acoustic impedance describes how the particles of a substance behave when subjected to a pressure wave
- Acoustic impedance also gives a measure of the resistance a substance has to the propagation of a sound wave through it
- A substance which has densely packed particles will have a high acoustic impedance
- A substance which has loosely packed particles will have a low acoustic impedance
- It is the acoustic impedance mismatch between two substances that determines the amount of energy reflected at an interface
- Soft tissue/air and soft tissue/bone interfaces produce strong reflections because of the large acoustic impedance mismatch between these substances. However, there is not enough energy transmitted to produce a useful image beyond these interfaces
- Ultrasound imaging is very good at discriminating between substances with small differences in acoustic impedance such as soft tissues

The ultrasound beam

5

CONTENTS

LEARNING OBJECTIVES

1 Describe the factors affecting the shape and uniformity of the ultrasound beam.

2 Explain the difference between beam width and slice thickness.

3 List the features of the ultrasound beam which can give rise to artifacts.

BEAM SHAPE

The area through which the sound energy emitted from the ultrasound transducer travels is known as the ultrasound beam. The beam is three-dimensional and is symmetrical around its central axis. It can be subdivided into two regions: a near field (or Fresnel zone) which is cylindrical in shape, and a far field (or Fraunhofer zone) where it diverges and becomes cone-shaped (see Fig. 5.1).

The actual shape of the beam depends on a number of factors, including the diameter of the crystal, the frequency and wavelength, the design of the transducer, and the amount of focusing applied to the beam. Increasing the frequency will result in a longer near field and less far field divergence. A narrow crystal diameter will result in a narrower beam in the near field, but the disadvantage is that the near field is shorter and there is more divergence in the far field.

Where there is continuous sound output from a transducer (primarily Doppler applications), there will be sound energy present throughout the beam for the duration of the scanning period. Most diagnostic applications, however, use pulsed sound, where the output is a series of short pulses of sound. In this case sound energy is not present

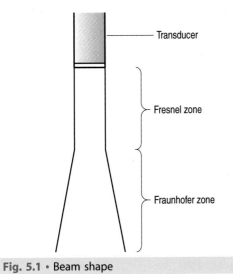

Fig. 5.1 • Beam shape

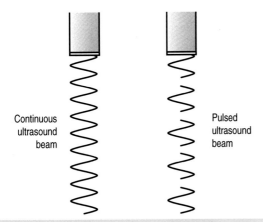

Fig. 5.2 • Pulsed and continuous wave ultrasound beam

throughout the beam, but only in small areas or pockets. It is the movement of these pockets of sound which we refer to as the ultrasound beam (see Fig. 5.2).

INTENSITY OF THE BEAM

The intensity of the beam is the power (measured in watts) flowing through a unit area (see Chapter 12 on Ultrasound safety). The intensity is not uniform throughout the beam's length nor across its width. This is caused by a number of variable factors such as:

- the beam does not have clearly defined edges and the intensity will decrease from the center outward
- the beam diverges which leads to the power distributing over a larger area in the far field
- interference effects exist in the near field from the numerous point sources of which the crystal is composed. A broadband transducer (see Chapter 6 on Transducers), due to its numerous frequency components, will show fewer interference effects and therefore more uniformity.

One noticeable result of the non-uniformity of intensity in the beam is that during scanning, a small reflector will give rise to a stronger echo if it is in the center of the beam (where there is maximum intensity of energy) than if it is on the periphery. This can therefore lead to a false interpretation by the operator as to the density of the reflector.

Where the beam is focused to improve spatial resolution, this will cause further non-uniformity of intensity, because a narrower beam will be created within the area known as the focal zone. The intensity is greatest in the focal zone and therefore a stronger echo will be received from a given structure that lies within the focal zone.

SIDE LOBES

Some of the energy from the transducer radiates at various angles to the transducer face, and these are known as side lobes. There may be one or more of these, and each of them will also be three-dimensional and will be the same frequency as the main lobe (see Fig. 5.3). Any interfaces encountered by

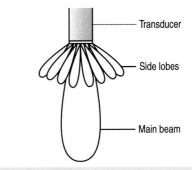

Fig. 5.3 • Side lobes

any of these side lobes will return echoes to the transducer, which the equipment erroneously assumes to have been received by the main beam. These echoes will therefore be incorrectly placed (or misregistered) on the image (see Chapter 9 on Artifacts). Approximately 15% of the energy in the beam will be within the side lobes. Manufacturers continually attempt to limit the amount of side lobes but are unable to eliminate them completely.

Array transducers will, in addition to the side lobes, also have grating lobes, which are lobes at various angles to the main beam. These only exist in the direction along which there are multiple elements within the array. Both side lobes and grating lobes can lead to considerable artifacts due to the three-dimensional misregistration which inevitably occurs. In addition, they cause a degradation of lateral resolution due to the effective widening of the beam in the scan plane.

BEAM WIDTH

Beam width refers to the dimension of the beam in the scan plane, or the plane through which the beam is sweeping (see Fig. 5.4). The actual beam width will vary according to the distance from the transducer, particularly where focusing is used. The width of each pulse of sound will therefore change with depth. The beam width affects the spatial resolution of the image (the ability of the operator to distinguish small structures) and generally, the narrower the beam width, the better the spatial resolution.

SLICE THICKNESS

The ultrasound image viewed on the monitor is a three-dimensional volume displayed as a two-dimensional image. The slice thickness refers to the dimension of the beam at 90° to the scan plane (see Fig. 5.4). Where the transducer has a circular crystal aperture, because the beam is symmetrical about its central axis, at any distance from the transducer, the beam width and slice thickness are equal. However, where transducers have rectangular apertures (phased array or linear array) the beam width and slice thickness can be very different. The slice thickness is usually larger than the beam width and cannot easily be reduced.

The fact that the beam width and the slice thickness are not finite results in artifacts occurring in the image (see Chapter 9 on Artifacts).

FOCUSING THE BEAM

The ultrasound beam can be focused, during both transmit and receive, to improve the quality within a particular zone of the image. This can be carried out in a number of ways (see Chapter 6 on Transducers) but the objective is to cause the beam to converge, which results in a narrowing of the beam (see Fig. 5.5). The operator can alter the depth of the focal zone or the number of focal zones. Increasing the number of focal zones will

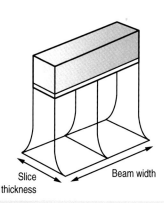

Fig. 5.4 • Beam width and slice thickness

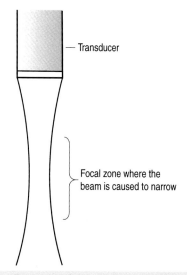

Fig. 5.5 • Focusing of the ultrasound beam results in narrowing of the beam

increase the size of the area with improved resolution, but will result in a slower frame rate of the image and poor temporal resolution (ability to visualize moving structures).

THE BEAM FORMER

An array transducer has multiple crystal elements (up to 128) and each has its own electrical connection to transmit the beam and receive the echoes. By manipulating the sequence of firing of these elements, the direction of propagation of the beam can be altered. This process is controlled by the beam former which can be manipulated by the operator. The beam former will control a variety of functions such as the focusing, beam steering, and switching between B mode and Doppler (see Chapter 6 on Transducers).

SUMMARY

- The ultrasound beam is three-dimensional and is symmetrical about its axis
- The shape of the beam depends on a number of factors, including the diameter of the crystal, the frequency and wavelength, the design of the transducer, and the amount of focusing applied to the beam
- The intensity of the beam is not uniform throughout its entire volume
- Inherent characteristics of the beam can lead to a number of artifacts such as side lobe artifacts, beam width artifacts, and slice thickness artifacts
- Manufacturers use a variety of technological features to optimize the beam, improve resolution, and reduce the artifacts

Transducers

CONTENTS

LEARNING OBJECTIVES

1 List the basic components that are used in the construction of a typical diagnostic ultrasound transducer.

2 Understand the operation of these devices.

3 Understand how ultrasound images are formed.

4 Explain how transducers can electronically focus and steer the ultrasound beam.

5 List the different types of electronic array transducers.

INTRODUCTION

The transducer is one of the most critical components of any diagnostic ultrasound system. There are many types of ultrasound transducers that can be selected before performing an ultrasound investigation as seen in Figure 6.1, and a great deal of attention should be paid to selecting the most appropriate transducer for the application.

Ultrasound transducers are described by their type and operating frequency which can range from 2 MHz up to 20 MHz and are selected based on their 'fitness for purpose'. The end user must recognize that different applications require an appropriately selected transducer which is best suited for a particular investigation.

We need to be aware that there is a trade-off between image resolution and the penetrating depth of ultrasound which is governed by its frequency. For example, a 12 MHz transducer has very good resolution, but cannot penetrate very deep into the body compared to a 3 MHz transducer which can penetrate deep into the body,

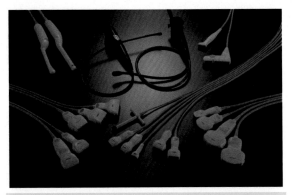

Fig. 6.1 • Ultrasound transducers (With permission from Toshiba Medical Systems.)

but the resolution is not as good as the transducer operating at 12 MHz. In general use, the highest frequency transducer which will reach the required depth should always be employed.

THE TRANSDUCER

Diagnostic transducers act as both a transmitter and receiver of ultrasound and are able to produce beams which can be directed in various ways to improve the quality of the images that we see on screen.

The primary component of the transducer is made from a piezoelectric material which means they are able to convert one form of energy to another, in this case electrical energy into mechanical energy and vice versa.

Components and Construction of a Typical Transducer

There are many types of transducers ranging from a simple single element to electronic multi-array probes which have hundreds of elements. The components and construction of these different types of transducers are principally the same. To understand how modern day electronic multi-element transducers function we need to start by considering the construction and components of a simple single element circular transducer. This is illustrated in Figure 6.2.

The main components of a typical ultrasound transducer consist of:

- physical housing assembly
- electrical connections
- piezoelectric element
- backing material
- acoustic lens
- impedance matching layer.

Physical housing

This contains all the individual components including the crystal, electrodes, matching layer, and backing material. This housing provides the necessary structural support and acts as an electrical and acoustic insulator.

Electrical connections

Two electrical connections are formed on the front and back face of the crystal by plating a thin film of gold or silver on these surfaces. These electrodes are connected to the ultrasound machine which

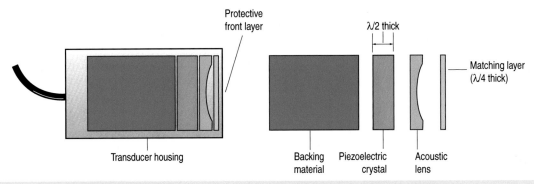

Fig. 6.2 • The construction and components of a simple single element circular transducer

generates the short burst of electrical pulses to excite the crystal and through the piezoelectric effect generates a pulse of ultrasound energy.

Piezoelectric element

Transducers operate on the piezoelectric effect which was discovered by Jacques and Pierre Curie in 1880. They found that certain crystalline minerals when subjected to a mechanical force became electrically polarized which means that they generated voltages. They also discovered that the converse was true, i.e. if a short electrical burst was applied to these crystals it would cause them to vibrate. The term 'piezoelectric' was derived from the Greek word 'piezein', meaning to press or squeeze.

By utilizing this piezoelectric property an ultrasound transducer can act both as a transmitter and receiver of ultrasound.

In transmission mode, a short burst of electric energy generated by the ultrasound scanner (typically one to three cycles of alternating voltage for imaging) is sent to the transducer generating an ultrasound pulse of energy. Reflected ultrasound echoes returning to the transducer face are detected, causing mechanical vibrations which are converted into electrical voltages. It is these electrical signals that are processed by the ultrasound machine which form the images that we see.

What are they made of?

Quartz is a naturally occurring material with piezoelectric properties and was extensively used in the development of early machines. This has now been superseded by man-made ceramics such as lead zirconate titanate (PZT) which are more efficient, have better sensitivity, and can easily be shaped.

How do you determine a transducer's operating frequency?

The operating frequency of a transducer is critically governed by the **thickness** of the piezoelectric crystal. For maximum efficiency the crystal should be operating at its 'natural' or 'resonant' frequency. This occurs when the thickness of the crystal corresponds to half a wavelength ($\lambda/2$).

We have already discovered that wavelength and frequency are inversely related, i.e. as wavelength decreases frequency increases, therefore we can appreciate that thinner piezoelectric materials produce higher resonant frequencies. Typical diagnostic ultrasound elements are between 0.2 mm and 1 mm thick.

A transducer operating at a resonant frequency of 2 MHz would have a thickness around 1 mm. In comparison, a transducer operating at a much higher frequency, say 7.5 MHz, would have a typical thickness of 0.3 mm.

Purpose of the backing material

Let us consider a simple single element transducer as illustrated in Figure 6.3. When a short burst or pulse of electricity is applied to a crystal it causes it to vibrate in all directions. The main vibrations come from the front and back faces of the piezoelectric crystal. We are only interested in the vibrations that come off the front face of the transducer. To try and eliminate the vibrations from the back face, and to control the length of vibrations from the front face, a backing or damping material is used. This damping material, which typically consists of tungsten powder and plastic or epoxy resin, is attached to the back face of the piezoelectric crystal.

Figure 6.4 shows that without the backing material a longer pulse of ultrasound is generated by a short burst of electricity as the crystal continues to vibrate or rings. These vibrations naturally fade out with time. An example of this effect can be heard when a cymbal is hit by a drumstick and continues to ring for some time. Attaching a backing material on the rear face of the element dampens the vibrations and generates a shorter ultrasound pulse. The length of the ultrasound pulse is known as the spatial pulse length (SPL).

Ultrasound pulses which are used for imaging are typically two to three cycles long. The advantage of having a short ultrasound pulse for diagnostic imaging is that it improves the resolution of the ultrasound images and in particular improves the **axial** resolution.

However, the damping material makes the generation of ultrasound less efficient and also reduces the sensitivity of the transducer to detect weak echoes. This is the price to pay for improved resolution.

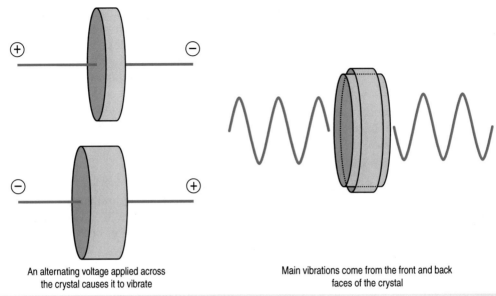

An alternating voltage applied across
the crystal causes it to vibrate

Main vibrations come from the front and back
faces of the crystal

Fig. 6.3 • When a short pulse of electricity is applied across the crystal it causes it to vibrate. The main vibrations are generated from the front and back face of the crystal

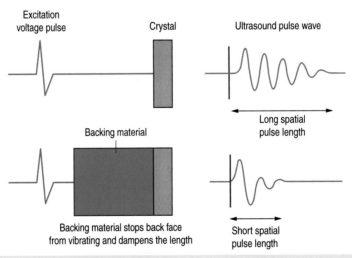

Excitation voltage pulse

Crystal

Ultrasound pulse wave

Long spatial pulse length

Backing material

Backing material stops back face from vibrating and dampens the length

Short spatial pulse length

Fig. 6.4 • The effect of a backing material is to eliminate any vibrations from the back face of the crystal and to produce a short pulse of ultrasound

Acoustic lens

The purpose of the acoustic lens is to improve image resolution by reducing the beam width of the transducer. The width of the beam determines the **lateral resolution**. The lateral resolution is the ability to resolve structures across or perpendicular to the beam axis. For a single element transducer sound may be focused by the addition of a lens

(Fig. 6.5a) or by using a curved piezoelectric crystal (Fig. 6.5b). The lateral resolution of an ultrasound beam varies with depth and is best at the focal region where the beam is narrowest.

Impedance matching layers

An acoustic impedance matching layer is sandwiched between the piezoelectric crystal and the

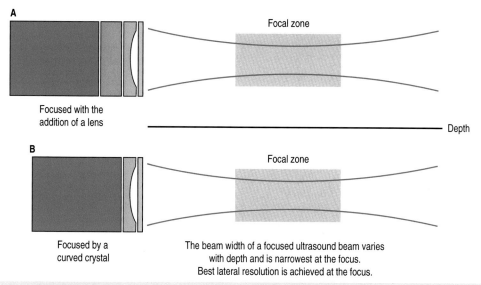

Fig. 6.5 · Focusing of the ultrasound beam achieved by a) utilizing a lens or b) using a curved piezoelectric crystal. Ultrasound beam is narrowest at the focal zone

patient and is an important factor that affects the sensitivity of the transducer, i.e. the ability of the ultrasound system to detect small reflected echoes. A large difference in acoustic impedance (Z) between two objects results in a large reflection of the incident ultrasound beam. The difference in acoustic impedance between the crystal and soft tissues within the patient is large (>15 times), and without this matching layer, most of the acoustic energy (typically 80%) would be reflected at this boundary with only around 20% being transmitted into the patient.

The matching layer typically has an acoustic impedance value halfway between that of the crystal and soft tissue. This results in more transmitted energy entering the patient and improves the signal strength of any returning echoes, which in turn improves the ultrasound system's sensitivity and image resolution.

More than one matching layer can be used and they are typically constructed to be one quarter wavelength thick ($\lambda/4$).

Relationship between Spatial Pulse Length and Bandwidth

We have discussed how transducers operate at their resonant frequency which is governed by the thickness of the piezoelectric crystal. However, the short pulses of ultrasound that are produced by damping the pulse in fact contain a range of frequencies which are centered around this operating frequency. The range of frequencies contained within an ultrasound pulse is referred to as its **bandwidth**. One of the factors that affect the bandwidth of a transducer is the spatial pulse length. Pulses which have short spatial pulse lengths contain a wider range of frequencies, i.e. have a wide bandwidth. On the other hand, ultrasound pulses which have longer spatial pulse lengths contain a narrower range of frequencies, i.e. have a narrow bandwidth. This is illustrated in Figure 6.6.

The wideband characteristics of modern day ultrasound transducers results in the end user being able to simply push a button to switch to a higher or lower operating frequency rather than changing the transducer. This enables the operator to choose a higher frequency to provide better detail resolution (resulting in some loss to the penetrating depth of the ultrasound beam) and switching to a lower frequency to increase the penetration of the ultrasound beam (resulting in some loss to image quality).

ELECTRONIC MULTI-ARRAY TRANSDUCERS

Electronic transducers have an array of rectangular shaped piezoelectric crystals etched side by side into one PZT ceramic (see Fig. 6.7a) which is

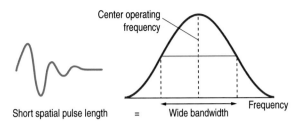

Center operating frequency

Short spatial pulse length = Wide bandwidth

Frequency

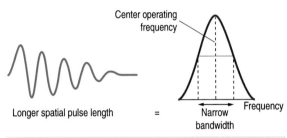

Center operating frequency

Longer spatial pulse length = Narrow bandwidth

Frequency

Fig. 6.6 • Demonstrating the relationship between spatial pulse length and bandwidth. The shorter ultrasound pulse contains a wider spread of frequencies known as the bandwidth. In comparison, a pulse which has a longer pulse duration, i.e. longer spatial pulse length, has a narrower bandwidth

mounted within the transducer housing. The internal components are similar to the simple single element transducer that was described earlier, in that they both have a backing material attached to the back face of the piezoelectric element to

shorten the pulse length, and matching layers attached to the front face to improve the sound transmission into the patient.

Typically, there are between 128–256 elements across the face of these transducers which are individually connected through one of the ultrasound machine ports. Figure 6.7b shows the hundreds of connections at the end of a transducer connector assembly.

Being able to control the firing sequence of each of the individual elements across the face of a transducer enables the operator, through the machine's front end controls, to manipulate the shape and direction of the ultrasound beam.

FORMING ULTRASOUND IMAGES

Ultrasound images are not created by firing all the elements in an electronic array transducer at the same time. They are formed by transmitting a series of small narrow beams along the transducer face which are directed along adjacent paths through the patient to generate one cross-sectional image.

Historically, early transducers were built to have one crystal which was moved mechanically by a small motor to sweep the beam over an area of the patient. An example of this early type of mechanical transducer is illustrated in Figure 6.8a which produces what is known as a sector field of view.

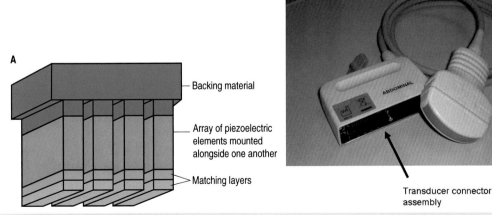

A
— Backing material

— Array of piezoelectric elements mounted alongside one another

— Matching layers

B

Transducer connector assembly

Fig. 6.7 • a) Internal construction components of an electronic array transducer. b) Picture of the hundreds of connections at the transducer connector assembly

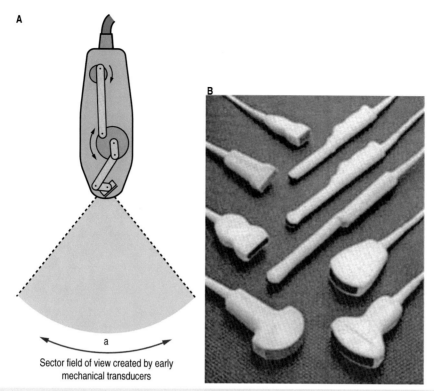

A

a

Sector field of view created by early
mechanical transducers

B

Fig. 6.8 • a) An example of an early mechanical transducer based on a single element which is mechanically swept over a range of angles to produce a sector field of view. b) A picture of a selection of modern day multi-element electronic transducers

Although these mechanical transducers can still be found, they were superseded by the modern electronic transducers that we use today (Fig. 6.8b).

Electronic transducers form an image by using small groups of elements (typically 5–10) to produce a narrow ultrasound beam which forms a scan line. The ultrasound machine can very rapidly sequentially sweep the position of this beam across the face of the transducer to produce a cross-sectional image as seen in Figure 6.9a. The firing sequencing of the groups of elements across a linear array transducer is illustrated in Figure 6.9b.

The first group of elements, in this case 1–5, are selected to create the first beam to form a scan line. Once all the returning echoes are received then a second group of elements are fired to form an adjacent scan line, again waiting for all the returning echoes to be received before moving onto the next group and so on. In this case this results in a rectangular image being produced for a linear array transducer.

ELECTRONIC BEAM FOCUSING AND STEERING

The ultrasound beam generated from electronic array transducers are formed by using groups of elements. These individual elements create small wavelets that interact with each other to form an overall ultrasound beam with a characteristic wavefront.

Consider a group of elements which are all excited simultaneously (seen in Fig. 6.10). The individual elements create small wavelets which interact together to form an ultrasound beam which has a wavefront that travels perpendicular to the face of the transducer.

By introducing a set of time delays to the individual elements, the ultrasound beam's shape

33

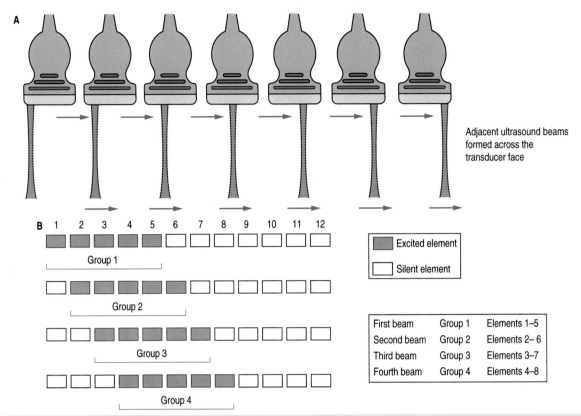

Fig. 6.9 • a) Ultrasound beam scanning is performed electronically by sequentially activating small groups of elements across the face of the transducer. b) Demonstrating the firing sequence for a group of elements across a transducer face

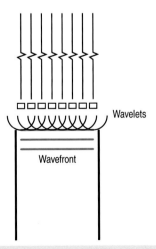

Fig. 6.10 • A group of elements are excited simultaneously, generating an ultrasound beam with a wavefront which travels perpendicular to the face of the transducer

and direction can be electronically manipulated to focus and steer the ultrasound beam.

Electronic Beam Focusing

We have already discussed that focusing the ultrasound beam improves the image quality (resolution) by making the beam thinner within the focal zone. A simple single element transducer focuses the beam by either utilizing an acoustic lens or by using a curved piezoelectric crystal. Electronic transducers focus the beam by introducing a series of time delays across a group of elements which are to be excited. Consider a group of nine elements which require a beam to be focused at a depth A (Fig. 6.11).

To create a beam which is focused at depth A requires all the wavelets created by each individual element to converge, i.e. to arrive at the desired

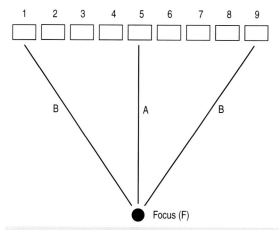

Fig. 6.11 • Path differences between the focal point and a group of elements

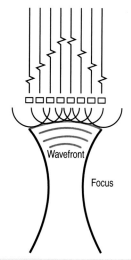

Fig. 6.12 • A typical sequence of time delays introduced across a group of elements to produce a focused ultrasound beam

focal point at the same time. We can see that the distance between the focus and the individual elements vary. The shortest distance is path A, between the focus and the center element. The longest distance, path B, involves the outermost elements (1 and 9). So to ensure that all the wavelets arrive at the same point at the same time, the ultrasound machine through the **beam former** introduces a set of time delays across the individual elements. As the outermost elements (1 and 9) have the furthest to travel they are excited first, followed by elements 2 and 8, then 3 and 7 and so on. The last element to be excited will be element 5. Figure 6.12 shows a typical sequence of time delays to produce an electronically focused beam.

Because focusing is achieved by introducing a set of electronic time delays, the position of the focal zone can be controlled by changing the timing sequence of these delays. Greater time delays create beams which are focused near to the transducer face. Longer time delays move the focal position further away from the transducer and deeper into the patient.

Operators are able to choose more than one focus and create beams with multiple focal zones which effectively creates a long narrow beam as illustrated in Figure 6.13. The advantage of using multiple focal zones is that overall image quality is improved throughout the image. The main disadvantage is that for each additional focal zone another pulse has to be sent out along the same

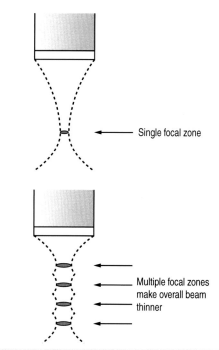

Fig. 6.13 • Effect of multiple focal zones on beam shape

Single focal zone

Multiple focal zones make overall beam thinner

scan line. The more focal zones selected the more time it takes to form a scan line which results in the frame rate being reduced, making the images appear disjointed.

Electronic Beam Steering

The ultrasound beam can also be steered by introducing a set sequence of time delays to the transmit pulses across a group of individual elements. The angle at which the beam is produced will depend on the delay between the excitation pulses of the individual elements. A typical sequence of time delays is demonstrated in Figure 6.14a. An image is formed by electronically sweeping the direction of the ultrasound beam across the transducer face by changing the delay between every set of excitation pulses so that the ultrasound beam is steered over a wide range of angles to form a wide 'sector' field of view (Fig. 6.14b).

TYPES OF ELECTRONIC ARRAY TRANSDUCERS

All the different types of transducers currently available can be characterized into three main types and are illustrated in Figure 6.15. They consist of:

- linear array transducers
- curvilinear (or sector) array transducers
- phased array transducers.

Linear Array Transducers

This type of array is typically made of between 128–256 elements in a row and produces parallel scan lines which are transmitted perpendicularly to the transducer face resulting in a rectangular field of view (see Fig. 6.15a). The width of this image is approximately equal to the length of the transducer head. Linear array transducers are used to image superficial structures and vessels and therefore operate at frequencies typically above 4 MHz. They are extensively used for vascular, small parts and musculoskeletal applications.

Curvilinear Array Transducers

This type of transducer is similar to a linear array but the transducer face is formed into a curve (convex in shape) which provides a wide field of view which diverges with depth (see Fig. 6.15b). These transducers are sometimes referred to as sector arrays. Curvilinear transducers operate at lower frequencies compared to linear arrays, typically around 3.5 MHz, and are best suited to image deep-lying structures. Their main applications are in abdominal and obstetric scanning.

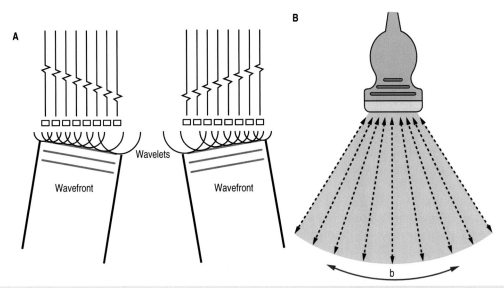

Fig. 6.14 • a) Typical time delay patterns introduced across a group of elements to steer the beam through a range of angles. b) Field of view created by beam steering

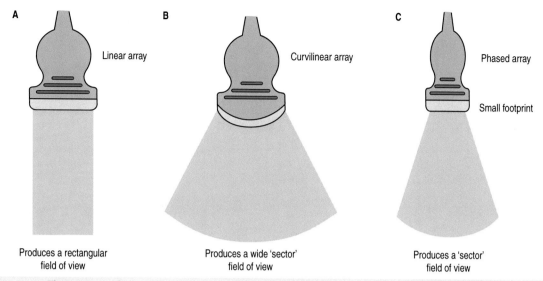

A Linear array

B Curvilinear array

C Phased array

Small footprint

Produces a rectangular field of view

Produces a wide 'sector' field of view

Produces a 'sector' field of view

Fig. 6.15 • Three types of electronic array transducers. a) Linear array; b) curvilinear array; c) phased array

Phased Array Transducers

Phased array transducers are similar to a linear array, being a flat-faced transducer with a row of elements positioned alongside one another. The crucial difference between the phased array and linear and curvilinear transducers is that the beam is **electronically steered** to produce an image. As a consequence of this, phased array transducers have a wide field of view similar to that of curvilinear transducers (see Fig. 6.15c).

These transducers are physically smaller than their counterparts and provide a wide field of view from a small transducer contact area, known as a footprint. The small footprint and wide field of view of these transducers are typically utilized in cardiac applications where it is difficult to image the heart because of the ribcage. These small transducers can easily fit between the ribs or underneath the ribcage to obtain an image of the heart. Typically operating at frequencies similar to curvilinear transducers, they are used to image deep-lying structures and perform specialized transcranial investigations.

SUMMARY

- Ultrasound transducers operate on the piezoelectric principle
- They convert electric energy into mechanical energy and vice versa; as a consequence of this they act as both a transmitter and receiver of ultrasound
- The thickness of the piezoelectric crystal determines the operating frequency
- The backing material shortens the ultrasound pulse length which improves axial resolution
- Focusing makes the ultrasound beam thinner, improving lateral resolution
- An ultrasound image is formed by sequentially sending out many adjacent ultrasound beams known as scan lines
- Modern day electronic transducers consist of an array of 128–256 elements that can be individually controlled by the beam former
- Electronic transducers can focus and steer the beam by introducing a sequence of varying time delays
- Common types of transducers include linear, curvilinear, and phased arrays

Resolution

7

CONTENTS

LEARNING OBJECTIVES

1 Define the term resolution as applied to an ultrasound image.

2 Explain what is meant by spatial, contrast, and temporal resolution.

3 Explain what is meant by axial and lateral resolution and list the factors affecting them.

4 Describe the factors that affect frame rate.

Resolution is a term which describes the ability of an imaging system to differentiate between structures, images, or events and display them as separate entities.

In this chapter we are going to examine the following categories of resolution and the factors that influence them:

- Spatial resolution – resolution in space
- Contrast resolution – resolution of gray shades
- Temporal resolution – resolution in time.

SPATIAL RESOLUTION

This is the ability to display two structures situated close together as separate images. When the structures are displayed as separate images we say that they are resolved (see Fig. 7.1).

In ultrasound imaging the spatial resolution depends ultimately on the wavelength of the sound used to produce the image. For example, the wavelength of a 5 MHz ultrasound beam is approximately 0.3 mm so it would not be possible to resolve objects less than 0.3 mm apart using a 5 MHz transducer.

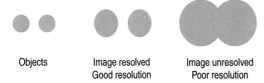

Fig. 7.1 • The difference between good resolution and poor resolution

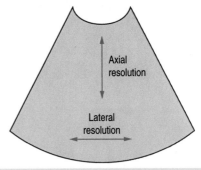

Fig. 7.2 • Axial resolution and lateral resolution on the image produced by a sector scanner

In ultrasound imaging, spatial resolution is divided into two components:

1 Axial resolution – resolution down the screen
2 Lateral resolution – across the screen (see Fig. 7.2).

Axial Resolution

This is resolution along the axis of the beam and depends upon the spatial pulse length – a short pulse length gives good axial resolution and the best resolution that can be achieved is half the spatial pulse length. For example if the pulse length is 1 mm then structures situated along the axis, which are less than 0.5 mm apart, will not be resolved (see Figs 7.3 and 7.4).

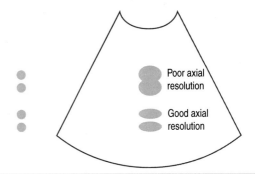

Fig. 7.3 • Poor axial resolution and good axial resolution

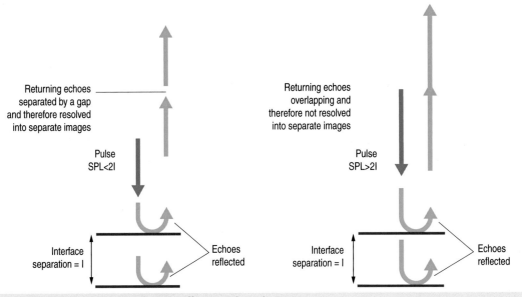

Fig. 7.4 • How spatial pulse length (SPL) affects axial resolution

Factors affecting spatial pulse length and therefore axial resolution

Frequency Each pulse of ultrasound is approximately two wavelengths long and therefore a shorter wavelength will reduce the pulse length. The wavelength of ultrasound depends on its frequency with the higher frequency waves having the shorter wavelengths. Therefore using ultrasound with a higher frequency for imaging will result in a shorter spatial pulse length and improved axial resolution.

Transducer design The pulse length depends upon the amount of damping applied to the piezoelectric crystal. The damping material is used to reduce 'ringing'; this is where the crystal continues to oscillate and produce sound after the driving voltage has ceased. Increasing the amount of damping makes the pulse length shorter and therefore improves the axial resolution.

Field of view (FOV)

Axial resolution may be affected by the FOV. In order for images of two structures to be resolved on the monitor screen they must be separated by at least 2 pixels, but as the FOV increases the distance represented by 2 pixels also increases. Therefore if the distance between the images of two structures is less than 2 pixels they will not be resolved.

The consequence of the above is that using a large FOV may be detrimental to the axial resolution (see Fig. 7.5).

Lateral Resolution

This is resolution at right angles to the beam and depends upon the beam width – a narrow beam width gives good spatial resolution and the best resolution that can be achieved is equal to the beam width at the focus of the beam (see Fig. 7.6).

The lateral resolution for a particular ultrasound machine is generally not as good as the axial resolution.

The beam width determines the size of the echoes displayed on the screen and structures must be separated by a distance greater than the beam width for them to be resolved into separate images (see Fig. 7.7).

Structures will only be resolved into separate images if the separation between them is greater

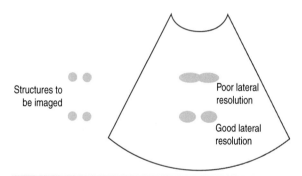

Fig. 7.6 • Poor lateral resolution and good lateral resolution

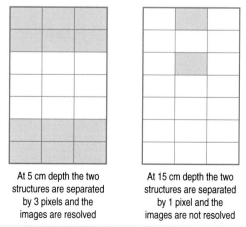

At 5 cm depth the two structures are separated by 3 pixels and the images are resolved

At 15 cm depth the two structures are separated by 1 pixel and the images are not resolved

Fig. 7.5 • How increasing the depth of the field of view may cause deterioration in axial resolution

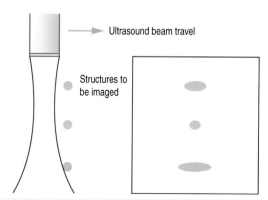

Fig. 7.7 • How beam width determines the size of the images displayed

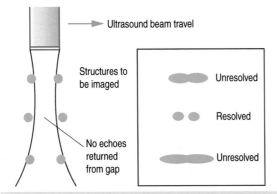

Fig. 7.8 • How structures must be separated by the beam width in order to be resolved into separate images

than the size of the beam width – the beam must fit into the gap between the two structures so that it can return 'no echoes' from that position (see Fig. 7.8).

Factors affecting beam width and therefore lateral resolution

Diameter of the piezoelectric crystal (aperture)

As the aperture increases the beam width close to the crystal face increases.

Transducer frequency Higher frequency beams have a longer near field and less divergent far field so the beam width is narrower than a lower frequency beam in these regions.

Focusing The degree of focusing, the length of the focal zone, and the number of focal zones all affect beam width.

Distance from the crystal (where lateral resolution is measured) The best lateral resolution is found at the focal point of the beam. The beam width increases the further it is from the focal point.

CONTRAST RESOLUTION

Contrast resolution is the ability of the imaging system to differentiate between body tissues and display them as different shades of gray. The main factors affecting it are as follows:

Transducer design Higher frequency transducers, which have a smaller slice thickness, generally provide better contrast resolution.

Analog to digital conversion This is a signal processing operation where the amplified voltage signal representing an ultrasound echo is converted into a binary number. During this operation there may be compression and filtering of the signal, which has an effect on the number of gray scales displayed and therefore the contrast resolution.

Control settings The following controls affect contrast and therefore the contrast resolution:

• Gain (amplification)
• Time-gain compensation (TGC)
• Post-processing and pre-processing options
• Harmonic imaging; this improves contrast
• Compound scanning. This improves edge definition but has a detrimental effect on contrast.

TEMPORAL RESOLUTION

This is the ability of the imaging system to display events which occur at different times as separate images. This is important when looking at rapidly moving structures such as the heart beating.

Temporal resolution is determined by the frame rate, which is the number of images displayed per second. The frame rate depends on a number of factors – these are illustrated in Figure 7.9.

Frame rate, pulse repetition frequency (PRF) and number of scan lines

The relationship between the frame rate, PRF and lines per frame is given by the following formula:

$$\text{frame rate} = \frac{\text{PRF}}{\text{lines per frame}}$$

Frame rate depends upon the PRF pulse repetition frequency and the number of scan lines per image:

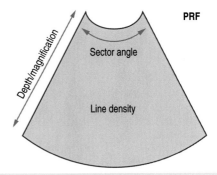

Fig. 7.9 • The factors affecting frame rate

Example

PRF = 1000 pulses per s
Number of lines per image = 100
Therefore frame rate = 10 frames per s

Factors affecting pulse repetition frequency

PRF depends upon image depth; an increase in image depth results in a lower PRF (see Fig. 7.10).

Factors affecting the number of lines per frame

The number of lines per frame depends upon the sector angle and the line density (lines per cm). An increase in either of these increases the number of lines per frame (see Fig. 7.11).

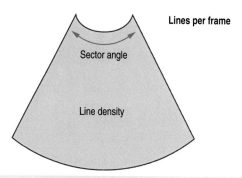

Fig. 7.11 • The factors affecting number of lines per frame

OPTIMIZING RESOLUTION

In order to optimize spatial resolution, the highest frequency, consistent with adequate penetration, should be selected. The ultrasound beam should also be focused at the area of interest and if movement of the subject is not a problem then multiple focal zones can be used.

To optimize contrast resolution, the highest frequency, consistent with adequate penetration, should be selected, together with the appropriate preset for the area being examined. Contrast is also optimized by using the correct overall gain and TGC settings.

Temporal resolution is improved by imaging at a high frame rate. This can be achieved by reducing the sector angle and depth to include only the area of interest and selecting a single focal zone.

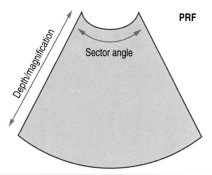

Fig. 7.10 • The factors affecting pulse repetition frequency

SUMMARY

- Spatial resolution is the ability of the imaging system to display two structures situated close together as separate images. When the structures are displayed as separate images we say that they are resolved
- Contrast resolution is the ability of the imaging system to differentiate between body tissues and display them as different shades of gray
- Temporal resolution is the ability of the imaging system to display events which occur at different times as separate images. This is important when looking at rapidly moving structures
- Resolution can be optimized by selecting a high frequency, consistent with adequate penetration, and appropriate adjustment of machine controls

Ultrasound interactions and attenuation

8

CONTENTS

LEARNING OBJECTIVES

1 Explain what is meant by the term attenuation.

2 Give the factors which influence attenuation.

3 Explain each of the interactions which are responsible for attenuation.

4 Describe how each of the above interactions affects the ultrasound image.

ATTENUATION

As the ultrasound beam travels through the body it loses energy. The **intensity** and **amplitude** of the sound wave decreases, and this process is known as **attenuation**.

The amount of attenuation that occurs will depend on the type of tissue the sound wave is traveling through. Where the molecules of the tissue are densely packed (such as bone), attenuation will be much greater than in less densely packed tissue (such as fat). Different tissues have different **attenuation coefficients** depending on the amount of attenuation occurring in the beam of sound.

Attenuation depends on the frequency of the sound. The higher the frequency, the greater the amount of attenuation that will occur in any given tissue.

Attenuation will occur not only in the beam of sound produced by the transducer as it propagates through tissue, but also in the returning echoes as they travel back to the transducer.

It therefore follows that returning echoes from deep within the patient will be of a much lower intensity than the initial beam of sound passing into the patient. It is for this reason that imaging equipment has a **time-gain compensation** (**TGC**) or depth-gain compensation (DGC) control, to allow for greater amplification of the weaker echoes returning from deeper within the body.

A variety of processes cause attenuation, but the five main processes to be considered are:

1 absorption
2 reflection
3 scattering
4 refraction
5 divergence.

Absorption

This is the main factor causing attenuation of the ultrasound beam. The higher the frequency of the sound wave, the greater the amount of absorption that will occur.

Energy is transferred from the sound wave into the medium through which it is traveling.

The rate of absorption depends on the **absorption coefficient** of the material through which it is traveling. Bone will have a much higher absorption coefficient than soft tissue. The absorption coefficient is proportional to the frequency. As an example, the absorption coefficient for a 7 MHz frequency wave is twice that of a 3.5 MHz frequency wave, e.g. a 3.5 MHz wave traveling through 1 cm of liver will have its intensity reduced by 50%, whereas a 7 MHz wave traveling through half this distance (0.5 cm of liver) will have its intensity reduced by the same amount.

Some absorption will be due to the energy lost from the sound wave in overcoming the opposition to its forward **propagation**. Other absorption will occur due to a transference of energy during the compressive part of the sound wave cycle.

The majority of the lost energy will cause a rise in temperature of the tissue through which the sound is traveling. This heating effect is a potential hazard when scanning biological tissue, although it can be used to advantage, for example, by physiotherapists when using ultrasound for treatment of soft-tissue injuries.

Reflection

As a beam of ultrasound travels through tissue it will encounter interfaces between different types of tissue. Where these interfaces are large compared with the size of the wavelength of the sound

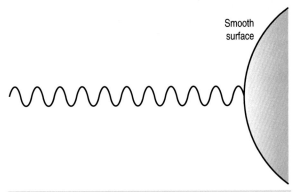

Fig. 8.1 • A large interface compared with the size of the wavelength of the sound

(such as organ boundaries (see Fig. 8.1)), some of the energy of the beam is reflected back in the form of an echo (see Fig. 8.2), while the remainder of the beam carries on traveling forward through the tissue. This is known as **specular reflection**.

The amount of energy that is reflected depends on the size of the **acoustic impedance mismatch** between the two tissue types. The greater the acoustic impedance mismatch, the greater the reflected component that occurs. At the interface between the liver and kidney, approximately 1% of the incident beam will be reflected. At the interface between the liver and biliary calculi, almost 40% is reflected, whereas at the interface between the liver and air in the bowel, 99.9% of the beam will be reflected. This, therefore, will result in very little information being transmitted beyond air or calculi, due to the large percentage of reflected sound. See Chapter 4 on Acoustic impedance.

The echoes reflected from large interfaces will only be returned to the transducer if the ultrasound

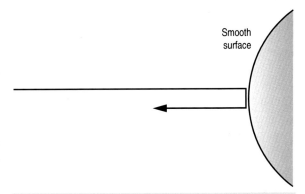

Fig 8.2 • Specular reflection from a smooth surface

beam is at 90° to the boundary. The angle of incidence of the ultrasound beam will always equal the angle of reflection (see Fig. 8.3). Any interfaces which are not perpendicular to the beam will, therefore, not be visualized during the scanning procedure, because the reflected echoes will not be received by the transducer.

Diffuse reflection

When the interface is rough and the undulations are approximately one wavelength or less (see Fig. 8.4) then sound is reflected in all directions. This is known as **diffuse reflection** (see Fig. 8.5).

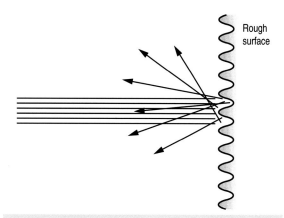

Fig 8.5 • Diffuse reflection

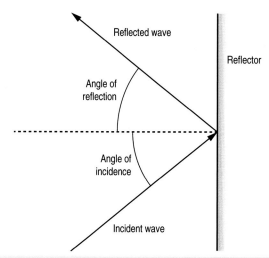

Fig. 8.3 • The angle of incidence and the angle of reflection are equal

Scattering

When an interface is equivalent to one wavelength in size, the reflected echoes are scattered in many directions (see Fig. 8.6). Because the wavelength depends on the frequency of the sound (the higher the frequency, the shorter the wavelength), more scattering will be noted at higher frequencies.

Some of this scattered energy will return to the transducer and be recorded as echoes. Organ parenchyma information will largely be composed of scattered energy (see Fig. 8.7). The majority, however, will be scattered non-uniformly in a variety of directions and not be recorded.

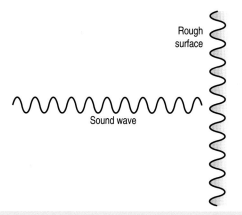

Fig. 8.4 • A rough interface with undulations equal to approximately one wavelength

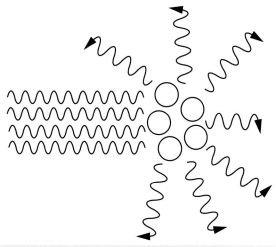

Fig. 8.6 • Interfaces that are approximately one wavelength in size and where the reflected echoes are scattered in many directions

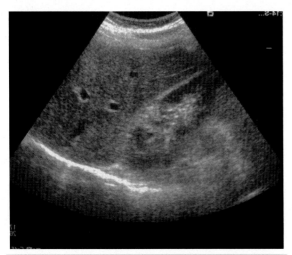

Fig. 8.7 • Image showing the effects of diffuse reflection and scatter from the parenchyma of the liver and specular reflection from the diaphragm and renal boundary

When an interface is smaller than the wavelength, the scatter is equal in all directions and is known as **Rayleigh scattering**.

Refraction

If a beam of sound passes through an interface between two tissues where the speed of sound is different, and if the angle of incidence is not perpendicular to the interface, then the path of the beam will be deviated or **refracted** (see Fig. 8.8). Both factors have to be present in order for refraction to occur, therefore, with an oblique angle of incidence between tissues of different acoustic impedances, no refraction would occur if the speed of sound were the same in both tissues.

Deviations of the beam of up to 10% may occur, and this can lead to incorrect placement or **misregistration** of displayed echoes (see Fig. 8.8). Some of this misregistration will appear as obvious artifacts; others may be more subtle and be wrongly interpreted by the operator. Errors in measurements can also result from this refraction of the beam. The actual amount of misregistration depends on both the size of the angle of approach, and the amount of difference in speed between the two tissues.

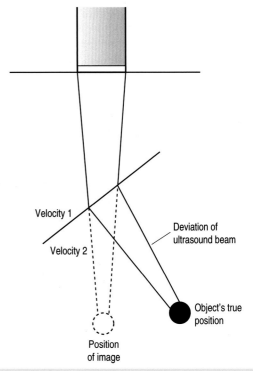

Fig. 8.8 • How a refracted ultrasound beam causes misregistration

Snell's law

This is a formula which gives the relationship between the angle of incidence and the angle of refraction when a beam of sound passes through an interface between two tissues where the speed of sound is different (see Fig. 8.9).

$$\frac{\sin\theta i}{\sin\theta r} = \frac{c_1}{c_2}$$

θi = angle of incidence

θr = angle of refraction

c_1 and c_2 = speeds of sound in the two media

Divergence

As a beam of ultrasound travels through tissue, it will diverge due to **diffraction** effects. This divergence will result in the same power spread over a larger area. The intensity (power/unit area) of the beam will therefore be reduced.

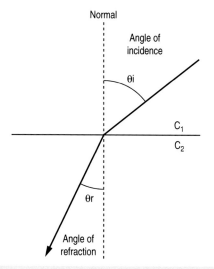

Fig. 8.9 • The variables in the Snell's law formula

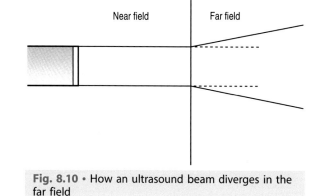

Fig. 8.10 • How an ultrasound beam diverges in the far field

In addition, the returning echo wave fronts will also diverge, causing a reduction in intensity with the greater the distance they travel.

Divergence will be most notable distal to the focal zone of a focused transducer or in the far field of a non-focused transducer (see Fig. 8.10).

SUMMARY

- As a sound wave travels through a medium, it loses energy, and as a result, its intensity and amplitude decrease, and it becomes attenuated
- Attenuation is proportional to the frequency of the sound wave and the distance that the wave travels
- The higher the frequency and the further the wave travels, the greater the attenuation
- In clinical imaging, the amount of expected attenuation should determine the frequency of the transducer that is selected
- When imaging a deep structure, a large amount of attenuation would be expected, therefore, a lower frequency transducer should be used
- Attenuation results from five main effects:
  - Absorption
  - Reflection
  - Scattering
  - Refraction
  - Divergence

Artifacts

9

CONTENTS

LEARNING OBJECTIVES

1 List the basic assumptions made by ultrasound equipment which gives rise to artifacts.

2 Describe the appearances of the more common artifacts encountered during ultrasound scanning.

3 Explain the causes of the commonly arising artifacts.

An ultrasound artifact is a structure in an image which does not directly correlate with actual tissue being scanned. Artifacts assume different forms, including:

- structures in the image that are not actually present
- objects that should be represented but are missing from the image
- structures which are misregistered on the image.

Where an operator is not aware of the presence of artifacts, it is possible that pathology will not be demonstrated and will therefore not be diagnosed (false negative result), or that pathology will be diagnosed where it does not exist (false positive result).

Understanding the basic mechanisms behind ultrasound artifacts, recognizing situations in which they are likely to arise, and becoming familiar with their appearance all help to eliminate misdiagnoses that may otherwise occur.

ASSUMPTIONS MADE BY ULTRASOUND EQUIPMENT

Ultrasound machines have to make certain assumptions in order to operate. These are:

- The speed of sound propagation is the same in all tissue types (usually equipment assumes this to be equal to 1540 m/s)
- The ultrasound beam travels in straight lines
- The time taken after emission of a pulse for an echo to return to the transducer from an interface is directly related to the distance of the interface from the transducer
- Attenuation of sound in tissue is uniform
- All echoes detected by the transducer have arisen from the central axis of the beam
- An echo generated at an interface returns directly in a straight line to the transducer without generating any secondary echoes
- The intensity or strength of the returning echo is proportional to the density of the reflector generating the echo.

These assumptions are often incorrect and will give rise to appearances which do not correspond to actual anatomy or tissue in the scan plane. It is these appearances that we term artifacts.

Several possible artifactual appearances may occur:

- There may be areas incorrectly showing absence of echoes
- Echoes may appear in areas which do not represent actual interfaces
- Separate structures may appear joined
- A single structure may appear as separate structures
- The brightness or textural appearance of echoes may not correlate with actual tissue structure
- Thin structures may appear thicker than reality or vice versa.

There are a multitude of different artifacts which may occur, but the more commonly occurring artifacts which will be discussed in this chapter are:

- reverberation
- acoustic shadowing
- acoustic enhancement
- edge shadowing
- beam width artifact
- slice thickness artifact
- side lobe artifacts
- mirror image
- double image
- equipment-generated artifacts.

REVERBERATION

This is the production of spurious (false) echoes due to repeated reflections between two interfaces with a high acoustic impedance mismatch. The echo from the interface is received by the transducer and displayed on the image. Some of the energy in the returned echo is reflected at the transducer face, and returns to the reflecting interface as if it was a weak transmitted pulse, returning as a second echo (reverberation). As the time taken for the second echo to arrive is twice that taken by the first echo, the image will display it at twice the depth. This sequence of reflection and transmission can occur many times, with the third echo taking three times as long to return to the transducer and being displayed at three times the depth, and so on. The reverberation echoes will be equally spaced because the time for each additional echo is a multiple of the time of return of the first echo. These reverberation echoes will be strong because of the high acoustic mismatch (see Fig. 9.1).

This artifact will often be seen:

- at the skin–transducer interface when the sound reverberates between the subcutaneous fat/muscle layer and the transducer (see Figs 9.2 and 9.3)
- behind bowel gas when the sound reverberates between the gas surface and the transducer (also known as ringdown) (see Fig. 9.4).

The artifact can be differentiated from real echoes due to the lack of breathing movement occurring.

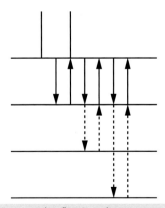

Fig. 9.1 • Repeated reflections between two interfaces cause reverberation of the displayed echoes

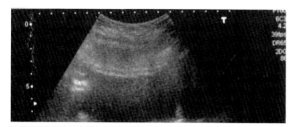

Fig. 9.2 • Reverberation occurring at the skin–transducer interface

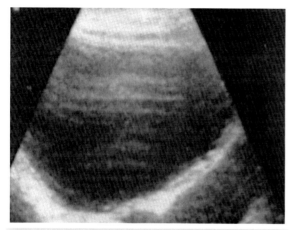

Fig. 9.3 • Reverberation arising at the skin–transducer interface and appearing in the bladder

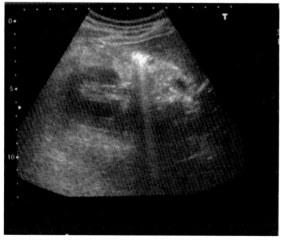

Fig. 9.4 • Reverberation occurring between bowel gas and transducer, appearing in the image distal to the bowel gas, and known as ringdown

To help to eliminate this artifact it may be useful to:

- increase the amount of gel used
- use a stand-off pad (such as a commercially produced gel pad or a bag of saline)
- reduce the gain
- move the position of the transducer.

ACOUSTIC SHADOWING

This appears as an area of low amplitude echoes (hypoechoic or anechoic) behind an area of strongly attenuating tissue. It is caused by severe attenuation of the beam at an interface, resulting in very little sound being transmitted beyond (see Fig. 9.5). The attenuation can be due to either absorption or reflection of the sound waves, or a combination of the two.

Acoustic shadowing will occur at interfaces with a large acoustic mismatch such as:

- soft tissue and gas (where the degree of attenuation will be due to reflection of 99.9% of the beam)
- soft tissue and bone or calculus (where the attenuation is due to a combination of approximately 40% reflection of the beam and 60% absorption by the bone).

It is often possible to differentiate diagnostically between structures such as gas in the duodenum or calculi in a small contracted gallbladder, by looking at the type of acoustic shadowing. Often shadowing in this area can be ambiguous and lead to an inaccurate diagnosis, but careful

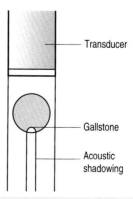

Transducer

Gallstone

Acoustic shadowing

Fig. 9.5 • Acoustic shadowing posterior to a strongly attenuating gallstone

examination will reveal different types of shadowing. If the shadowing contains reverberation (ringdown) echoes, it is likely to be gas (see Fig. 9.6a & b). If the shadowing is clear shadowing, absent of any ringdown, it is likely to be a calculus (see Fig. 9.7 a & b).

ACOUSTIC ENHANCEMENT

This artifact appears as a localized area of increased echo amplitude behind an area of low attenuation. On a scan it will appear as an area of increased brightness, and can commonly be

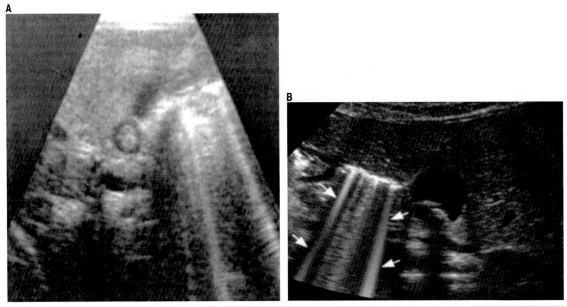

Fig. 9.6a & b · Acoustic shadowing occurring in the region of the gallbladder (suggesting possible biliary calculi), but as it contains ringdown, it is more likely to be caused by gas in the adjacent bowel

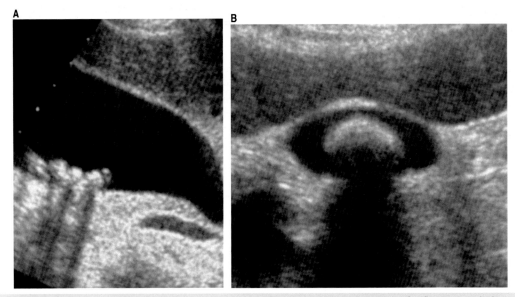

Fig. 9.7a & b · Acoustic shadowing posterior to biliary calculi due to a combination of reflection and absorption

seen distal to fluid-filled structures such as the urinary bladder, the gallbladder, or a cyst.

The artifact arises due to the application of the time-gain compensation (TGC) to areas of low attenuating structures such as fluid. It is caused by the low level of attenuation of the beam as it passes through fluid relative to the greater attenuation of the beam in the adjacent more solid tissue (see Fig. 9.8). As the echoes pass beyond the area, they will be of higher amplitude than the surrounding tissue because they have been amplified unnecessarily. The high amplitude brightness therefore does not relate to any inherent scattering or reflectivity properties of the tissue, but arises because the equipment assumes a uniform rate of attenuation across the entire image (see Fig. 9.9).

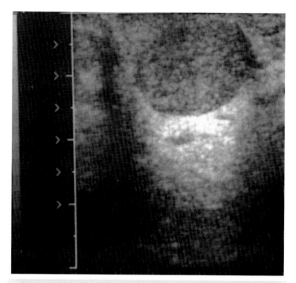

Fig. 9.10 • Acoustic enhancement posterior to a soft tissue mass

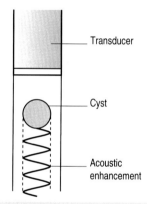

Fig. 9.8 • Acoustic enhancement posterior to a low attenuating cyst

This artifact can often be a useful diagnostic aid, particularly when scanning a soft-tissue mass or cyst containing low-level echoes. These echoes may often cause the structure to disappear in the image as it blends into the surrounding echo pattern. The observant operator will often notice the echo enhancement, resulting in a closer examination of the area above this, and the mass or cyst will then be delineated (see Fig. 9.10).

EDGE SHADOWING

A combination of refraction and reflection occurring at the edges of rounded structures (and when the speed of sound is different from that in surrounding tissue) will result in an edge shadowing artifact.

Edge shadowing arises due to refraction of the beam caused by both the curvature of the rounded edges and the difference in speed of the two materials. When the ultrasound beam reaches the rounded edge of a structure, reflection will occur, with the angle of incidence equal to the angle of reflection. The outer part of the beam will be totally reflected, but the remainder of the beam passes through the rounded structure and is refracted (deviated from its original path) (see Fig. 9.11). This combination of reflection and

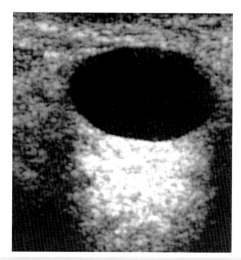

Fig. 9.9 • Acoustic enhancement posterior to a cyst

55

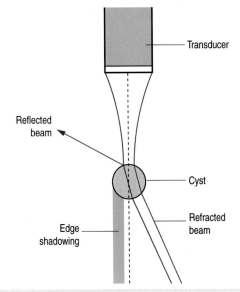

Fig. 9.11 • Edge shadowing

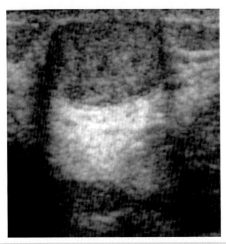

Fig. 9.13 • Edge shadowing posterior to a soft-tissue mass

refraction of the beam at the edge of a rounded structure results in a thin strip of tissue behind the edge not being insonated and causes a shadow. These shadows are narrow and occur directly distal to the margins of the rounded structure, such as either a cyst (see Fig. 9.12) or a soft-tissue mass (see Fig. 9.13). The shadowing should normally be readily identified as an artifact, however it is possible that it may be falsely diagnosed as areas of calcification within an organ.

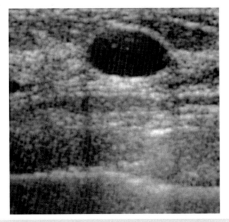

Fig. 9.12 • Edge shadowing posterior to a cyst

BEAM WIDTH ARTIFACT

All the echoes returning to the transducer will have arisen from across the full width of the beam, which can vary by several millimeters. As the beam sweeps through the patient, a point reflector will generate an echo for as long as it remains in the beam, and the reflector will be represented as a line in the display rather than a dot. The length of the line will therefore represent the beam width at that depth. This artifact can be demonstrated by scanning a point reflector in a phantom, where the display will clearly portray this as a line (Fig. 9.14).

During routine scanning, the artifact can be seen when spurious echoes are displayed in an echo-free area, for example when reflections from bowel are generated by the edge of the beam and displayed inside the sagittal view of the urinary bladder, where the center of the beam is (see Figs 9.15 & 9.16).

Correct positioning of the focal zone will help to reduce this artifact. The focal zone is controlled by electronically narrowing the beam (see Chapter 5 on The ultrasound beam).

SLICE THICKNESS ARTIFACT

These occur due to the thickness of the beam, and are similar to beam width artifacts (see Chapter 5 on The ultrasound beam). However, they occur at 90° to the scan plane (see Fig. 9.17), with echoes from interfaces in front of and behind the assumed plane of origin appearing in the display.

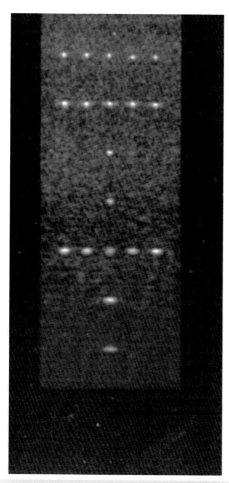

Fig. 9.14 • Scan of a phantom demonstrating that the point reflectors can be seen as points in the center of the image where the focal zone is set (and the beam is therefore narrowest), but the same points appear as lines where they lie outside the focal zone (and the beam is wider)

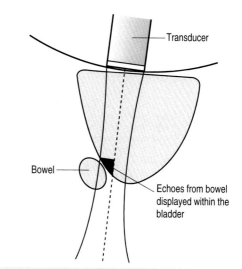

Fig. 9.15 • Beam width artifact

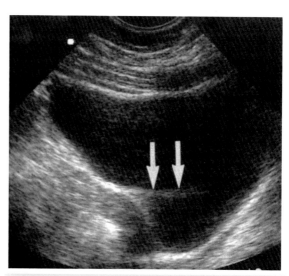

Fig. 9.16 • Beam width artifact in a sagittal view of the bladder

It is assumed that the echoes detected by the transducer are from a very thin slice of tissue. However, the reality is that this slice is actually composed of several slices of information and therefore echoes from interfaces on either side of the intended thin slice will be included in the displayed image (see Fig. 9.18). Increasing the slice thickness will increase the number of artifactual echoes in the display.

These artifacts will typically be seen in transverse views of the urinary bladder when structures adjacent to the slice through the bladder being scanned will be incorporated into the image. These echoes are then displayed as if they were arising from within the bladder (see Fig. 9.19). Although the appearance of this artifact is similar to the beam width artifact, the differentiating factor is that the reflector causing the slice thickness artifact will not be seen on the display.

This artifact is a result of inherent characteristics of the transducer, and apart from trying a different transducer, cannot be eliminated. New technology, however, is continuously resulting in narrower slice thicknesses.

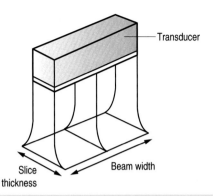

Fig. 9.17 • Beam width and slice thickness

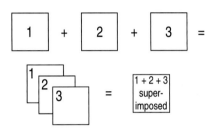

Fig. 9.18 • Each image is composed of several slices of information added together

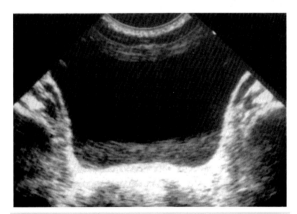

Fig. 9.19 • Slice thickness artifact in a transverse view of the bladder

SIDE LOBE ARTIFACT

The energy within the ultrasound beam exists as several side lobes radiating at a number of angles from a central lobe (see Fig. 9.20). Echoes are generated by these side lobes in addition to the main lobe, but all the returning echoes are assumed by the

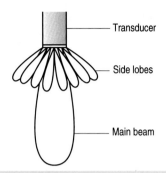

Fig. 9.20 • Side lobes

transducer to have arisen from the central axis of the main lobe (see Chapter 5 on The ultrasound beam). Side lobe echoes will therefore be misregistered in the display. Because ultrasound beams are three-dimensional, side lobes exist not only in the scan plane but also in the entire 360° around the beam. The echoes generated by the side lobes are usually much lower in amplitude than the main beam and will therefore often not be seen, unless the echoes are returning from a strong reflector such as gas.

This artifact can often be seen in areas such as the urinary bladder where the side lobes detect echoes from adjacent bowel and the equipment registers these echoes as if they have arisen from within the bladder. They may also arise within a cyst, where adjacent structures are portrayed as if arising from within the cyst (see Fig. 9.21). These appearances can give rise to a false diagnosis of septations within a cyst.

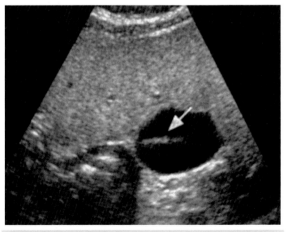

Fig. 9.21 • Artifact in a cyst caused by information obtained by the side lobes and leading to possible misdiagnosis of a septated cyst

MIRROR IMAGE ARTIFACT

These artifacts result in a mirror image of a structure occurring in an ultrasound display. They arise due to specular reflection of the beam at a large smooth interface. An area close to a specular reflector will be imaged twice, once by the original ultrasound beam and once by the beam after it has reflected off the specular reflector. Echoes return along the same path from the reflecting interface, back to the transducer. Because the equipment assumes all echoes arise from a straight beam, the reflected echoes are displayed in a line as if originating from below the specular reflecting surface (see Fig. 9.22).

Mirror image artifacts are most commonly seen where there is a large acoustic mismatch, such as a fluid–air interface. Typically this artifact can occur during the scanning of a full urinary bladder, when air in the rectum behind the bladder acts as a specular reflector and a mirror image of the bladder is displayed posteriorly. It will then have the appearance of a large cyst behind the bladder (see Fig. 9.23). It can also be seen when scanning the liver, and the diaphragm acts as a specular reflector. In this case the liver parenchyma is displayed not only below the diaphragm but also above it (see Fig. 9.24). When trying to determine whether these appearances represent pathology or artifact, it is important to recognize whether the echoes have the same appearance as the organ from which they have arisen.

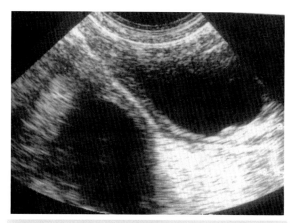

Fig. 9.23 • Mirror image artifact of the bladder imitating a cyst in the pelvis

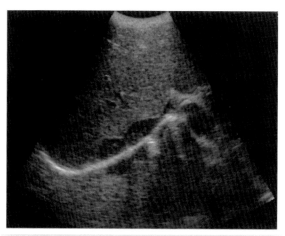

Fig. 9.24 • Mirror image artifact of the liver appearing above the diaphragm (From Bates 1999, with permission of Churchill Livingstone.)

DOUBLE IMAGE ARTIFACT

This artifact is caused by refraction of the beam and may occur in areas such as the rectus abdominis muscle on the anterior abdominal wall. In the transverse plane the edges of the muscle act as a lens and cause the ultrasound beam to be refracted (i.e. deviated from its original path) and this causes a single structure to be interrogated by two separate refracted beams (see Fig. 9.25). Two sets of echoes will therefore be returned and these will cause display of two structures in the image. This results in, for example, two images of the transverse aorta side by side in the abdomen (see Fig. 9.26). Alternatively, a single gestation sac can

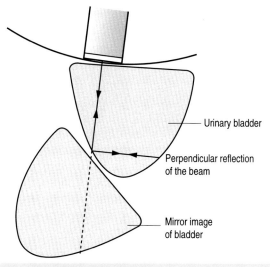

Urinary bladder

Perpendicular reflection of the beam

Mirror image of bladder

Fig. 9.22 • Mirror image artifact

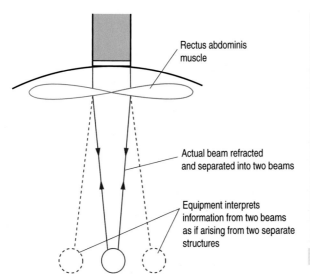

Rectus abdominis muscle

Actual beam refracted and separated into two beams

Equipment interprets information from two beams as if arising from two separate structures

Fig. 9.25 • Double image artifact caused by refraction of the beam

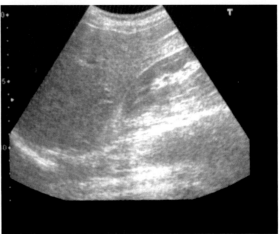

Fig. 9.27 • Too much gain causing artifactual echoes

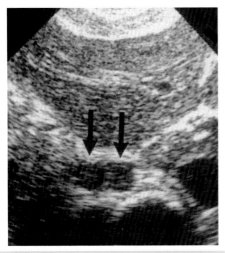

Fig. 9.26 • Double image artifact of the aorta

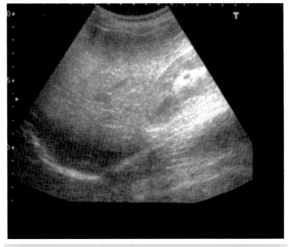

Fig. 9.28 • Incorrect use of TGC causing artifactual echoes

be mirrored and appear as two gestation sacs side by side, leading to the erroneous diagnosis of a twin pregnancy. In order to establish whether these echoes are genuine, it is necessary to move the transducer slightly to one side to avoid the junction of the rectus abdominis muscles.

EQUIPMENT-GENERATED ARTIFACTS

Incorrect use of the equipment controls can lead to artifacts appearing. Misuse of controls such as the gain (see Fig. 9.27) or TGC (see Figs 9.28 & 9.29)

can result in echoes being recorded as too bright or too dark. Care must be taken when setting these controls, to ensure an even brightness throughout the image. If too much gain is applied then the electronic noise, inherent in all systems, will also be amplified. This has the appearance of a fine overlay of low-level echoes in the image and will cause deterioration of the quality of the image, reducing the ability of the operator to correctly interpret. If too little gain is applied, this can lead to loss of relevant information, and incorrect diagnosis may occur.

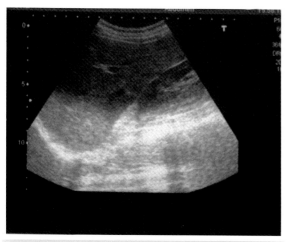

Fig. 9.29 • Incorrect use of TGC causing artifactual appearances

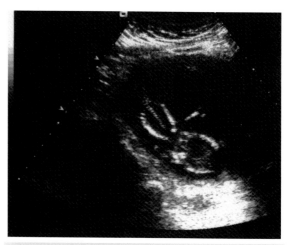

Fig. 9.30 • The image has too much contrast resulting in the loss of subtle information

If the dynamic range control is incorrectly set, this can lead to an image which has too much contrast, and result in the loss of subtle echo information (see Fig. 9.30).

Blurring of a moving image can occur if the frame rate is too low or if the persistence is too high. It is important to ensure that the frame rate is capable of recording a moving structure at the correct speed.

Use of multiple focal zones can give rise to a prominent banding effect within the image. These are usually identifiable as being of electronic origin due to the well-defined margin of the bands.

SUMMARY

- An ultrasound artifact is a structure in an image which does not directly correlate with actual tissue or structures
- Artifacts occur due to false assumptions made by the equipment
- Failure to recognize artifacts can lead to misdiagnosis
- Many different artifacts occur during routine ultrasound scanning but the more common ones include:
  - Reverberation
  - Acoustic shadowing
  - Acoustic enhancement
  - Edge shadowing
  - Beam width artifact
  - Slice thickness artifact
  - Side lobe artifact
  - Mirror image
  - Double image artifact
  - Equipment-generated artifacts

Reference

Bates JA 1999 Abdominal ultrasound, 2nd edn. Churchill Livingstone, Edinburgh.

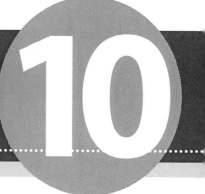

Instrumentation and controls

CONTENTS

LEARNING OBJECTIVES

1 List the primary components of an ultrasound machine.

2 Understand the basic function of each component.

3 Identify the primary operator-dependent controls.

4 Explain how a number of key controls influence image quality.

INTRODUCTION

A diagnostic ultrasound machine consists of many components, each of which has a separate operation to perform. This starts with transmitting and receiving ultrasound signals which are then processed to form the images that we see on screen. The internal components that make up a typical ultrasound machine are listed below. Figure 10.1 illustrates the architecture of the components in a block diagram.

- Transducer
- Pulser
- Beam former
- Receiver
- Processor
- Display
- Digital storage
- Hard copy printer devices.

COMPONENTS OF A TYPICAL ULTRASOUND MACHINE

The Transducer

Diagnostic transducers are made from piezoelectric materials (see chapter on Transducers) and

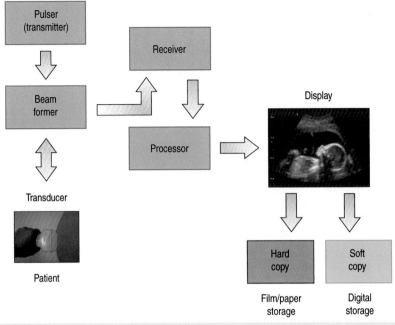

Fig. 10.1 • A block diagram of an ultrasound imaging machine

are able to convert electrical energy into ultrasound energy and vice versa. As a consequence of this they can act as a transmitter and receiver of ultrasound. They are able to produce beams which can be directed in various ways which are controlled by the ultrasound machine to improve image quality.

The Pulser

The pulser produces the electric voltage that drives the transducer. This driving voltage governs the output power of the ultrasound machine and can be adjusted by the operator through the power or output control. Changes in the applied voltage to the transducer changes the strength and intensity of the ultrasound beam, and affects the overall brightness of the B-mode image. The greater the applied voltage, the stronger the ultrasound pulse and the higher the pulse intensity. Figure 10.2 illustrates the effect that increasing the applied voltage has on the B-mode image. Increasing the applied voltage to the transducer increases the ultrasound pulse intensity, resulting in an increase in the overall brightness of the image.

Beam Former

The beam former controls the shape and direction of the ultrasound beam and the scanning patterns used to form the images that we see. This enables the operator to have indirect control of:

- depth
- focus
- sector width
- zoom.

Receiver

The job of the receiver is to combat attenuation, i.e. the energy lost from the beam as it propagates through soft tissue. As a consequence of attenuation the returning echo amplitudes and intensities are decreased. Most of the energy is lost from the beam through absorption which is mainly converted into heat. The receiver applies amplification to the returning echoes to make them stronger and to enable them to be visualized. The ultrasound machine can compensate for the effects of attenuation by amplifying the received signals in two ways, using the overall gain and the time-gain compensation (TGC) controls.

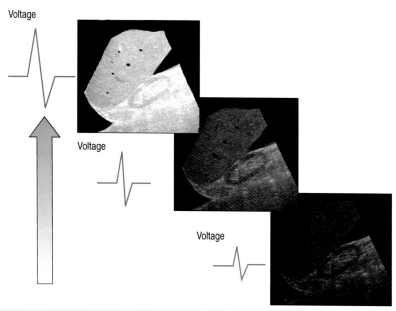

Fig. 10.2 • Increasing the applied voltage to the transducer increases the pulse intensity and output power, resulting in brighter images

Processor

The processor can be divided into two individual parts, each having very different tasks to fulfil, and consists of:

- a signal processor – converts echo voltages to video signals
- an image processor – formats the many scan line data into image form.

A simple block diagram of the **signal processor** is illustrated in Figure 10.3. The signal processor

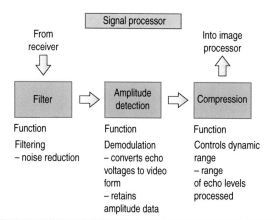

Fig. 10.3 • Block diagram of the signal processor outlining the key functions of each component

picks up the amplified signals from the receiver and carries out operations such as filtering, amplitude detection, and signal compression.

Filtering cleans up the signal, removing unwanted noise, and also controls the signal bandwidth (see chapter on Transducers). Amplitude detection performs a process of demodulation which means it converts the received signal voltages into video form, retaining the amplitude information required for B-mode imaging. Compression controls the dynamic range of the B-mode image (the number of shades of gray displayed in the image).

Once the signals have passed through the **signal processor** they are fed into the image processor. A block diagram of the image processor is illustrated in Figure 10.4. The image processor performs operations such as scan conversion which reformats the scan line data into two-dimensional images, i.e. either linear or sector form. The ability of the scan converter to rapidly process the thousands of scan line data received every second from the transducer enables real-time dynamic ultrasound imaging to be performed.

There is a range of processing performed on the image data prior to and following storage into memory before they are finally sent to the display. Functions such as edge enhancement are known as

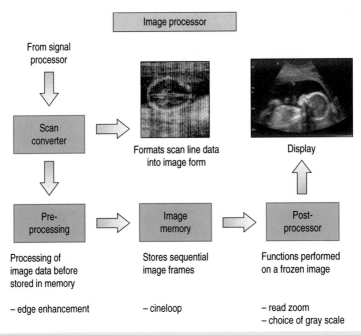

Fig. 10.4 • A block diagram of the image processor outlining the key functions of each component

pre-processing functions because they are performed before being stored.

Image memory stores a number of sequentially acquired and processed static image frames every second which are rapidly sent to the display to provide dynamic real-time ultrasound. This process can be interrupted by activating the freeze control which stops any further acquisition and processing of data from the transducer. In freeze mode only one static image in the memory is displayed. The numerous frames of image data held and stored can be reviewed in turn using the machine's cineloop control function.

The Display

Once the images have been processed they can either be displayed on a traditional cathode ray tube which is used in conventional televisions or be presented on a computer monitor or a flat panel screen. There are only two controls that can be adjusted on most displays, which are brightness and contrast. These can be set by the operator according to individual preference or ambient room lighting conditions.

Hard Copy and Soft Copy Storage

The images displayed on screen can be sent out to an external hard copy device such as radiographic film or thermal paper printers. Alternatively, the images, which can also consist of short cineloop review video clips, can be digitally stored on the machine's hard disc or alternatively burnt to CD or DVD. Many ultrasound departments are linked into a picture archiving and communications system, more commonly known as PACS. This enables images such as X-rays and ultrasound scans to be stored electronically and viewed on any PACS display monitor around the hospital at the touch of a button.

SYSTEM CONFIGURATION – USE OF PRESETS

Many ultrasound machines provide the operator with a range of stored preconfigured control settings known as presets. Before starting any investigation the operator should select and initialize the specific preset which has been configured to automatically select various control parameters such as gain, depth, power, focus, etc., together with the most appropriate processing functions to optimize the image performance of the ultrasound system. There are a number of different presets which can be selected by the operator for each type of clinical examination whether it be, for example, liver, pelvis, obstetric, abdominal, or vascular. The ultrasound system can also store additional presets for different users; each stored preset can be selected with a single keystroke.

Despite the inclusion of system configured presets in most current ultrasound equipment it is important for the operator to have an understanding of the function of each manual control, because many of these preset modes will require further manual manipulation throughout the scanning procedure. Patient body habitus will vary significantly, resulting in a requirement for changes to the equipment controls throughout the examination.

FUNCTION OF ULTRASOUND CONTROLS

Image Controls

A large number of controls are available to be used on most ultrasound equipment but the more important and most frequently used controls are discussed below.

Output power

The output power of an ultrasound machine is determined by the pulser which produces the electric voltage that drives the transducer. The output power is automatically set for each preset mode and can be manually manipulated through the power or output control. Ultrasound machines' output powers are limited, and should not exceed $720 \, \mathrm{mWcm}^{-2}$ specifically for safety reasons (see chapter on Ultrasound safety).

The effect of increasing the output is to increase the amplitude and intensity of emitted ultrasound pulses which in turn increases the size of the returning signals. Improving the signal strength of returning echoes improves the clarity and detail of structures within the B-mode image. The effect of increasing the output power is demonstrated in Figure 10.2 which shows that the higher the output power, the brighter the overall B-mode image.

However, increasing the output power causes the patient to be exposed to more ultrasound energy which could increase the risk of causing any possible harmful effects that are more likely to affect sensitive tissues such as rapidly developing cells found in embryo, fetus, and neonate. The alternative and safer option rather than increasing the output power is to amplify the received signals using the machine's gain and/or TGC controls. This minimizes exposure while improving the image quality.

Overall gain

Overall receiver gain provides uniform amplification of all the received signals regardless of depth, and affects the brightness of the overall image. The operation of the gain is to compensate for the loss of energy through attenuation as the beam propagates through the patient.

There is no 'absolute' or 'correct' setting. The gain will require adjustments throughout the examination and will vary with each individual patient according to the organ or vessel being scanned or to the body habitus of the patient. This will involve increasing the level of the gain for scanning deeper structures and decreasing it when scanning superficial structures. However, there is a limit to how much the received signals can be amplified which is governed by the level of noise within the signal.

Amplifying the signal strength also amplifies the level of background noise within the signal, which becomes more significant as the levels of amplification increase to the point where the level of the background noise in the signal is greater than that of the received signal. The depth at which this occurs is known as the penetration depth. When background noise is visualized this is the point to stop increasing the gain and to increase the output power if safe to do so.

Time-gain compensation (TGC)

The TGC is similar to the overall gain inasmuch as they both compensate for the effects of attenuation. Attenuation causes weaker signals to be received from structures that lie deeper than those which lie closer to the face of the transducer. The TGC can compensate for this loss of signal strength so that equal amplitudes can be

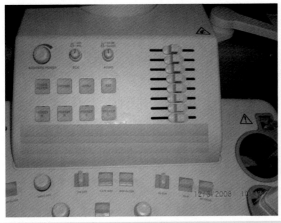
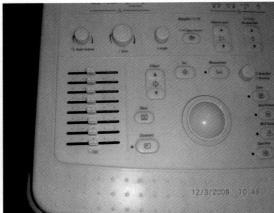

Fig. 10.5 • Examples of TGC slider controls

displayed from all depths within the scan plane as the same brightness on the image. This is simply achieved by applying a variable gain to the received signals so that signals returning later are amplified more than those previously received. The TGC does this through a number of horizontal slider controls as shown in Figure 10.5. Their relative position governs the amount of gain applied to the received signals from various depths within the scan plane. The net result produces received signals of similar amplitude and displayed brightness over depth.

The processes involved with TGC of received signals are illustrated in Figure 10.6.

Depth

The depth control changes the maximum scanning range viewed on screen. The ultrasound machine determines depth indirectly by measuring the time

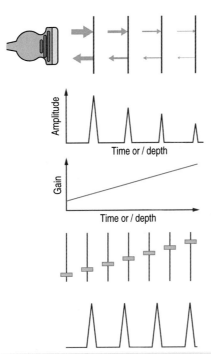

A. Transducer receives returning echoes from different depths (times) from similar boundaries.

B. Attenuation causes weaker signals to be received from boundaries that lie deeper than those which lie closer to the transducer.

C. To compensate for this effect a variable gain is applied which increases with the time that the signals are received.

D. The TGC slider controls are adjusted by applying sloping of the TGC throughout the image.

E. The net result produces received signals with similar amplitude and displayed brightness

Fig. 10.6 • Illustrating the processes involved with TGC of received signals (After Thrush & Hartshorne 2005.)

it takes for a pulse to return. The system has to wait to receive all the returning echoes along each scan line for a selected depth before sending another. As the depth control is increased the time it takes for a pulse to return to the transducer also increases. This time factor imposes an upper limit to the time interval between consecutive transmit pulses known as the pulse repetition frequency (PRF). Changes in the depth changes the maximum pulse repetition rate which affects the frame rate.

Increasing the depth decreases the system's PRF which decreases the number of image frames that can be displayed per second (fps).

Focus

The focus determines the depth at which the ultrasound beam is focused and creates the best possible resolution at that depth.

The focal position is usually displayed by a symbol or vertical bar or bracket alongside the display of the B-mode image. The focal zone should be positioned at or just below the level of interest within the B-mode image. The operator is able to activate more than one focal zone, sometimes as many as five, however for each additional focal zone another pulse must be sent along the same scan line. As a consequence of this, the number of frames of image data per second (fps) is reduced, resulting in a slower frame rate and the images appearing disjointed.

The number of focal zones is related to the frame rate and is illustrated in the example below:

Example

Consider a B-mode image which is made up of 100 scan lines of data. With 100 lines per image:

Using	1 focal zone	40 fps can be achieved
	2 focal zones	20 fps
	3 focal zones	10 fps
	4 focal zones	2 fps

Doubling the number of focal zones halves the frame rate

Freeze and cineloop

Activating the freeze button stops any further acquisition and processing of data from the transducer. Once frozen the ultrasound machine displays the last acquired image which is held in image memory. Image memory is able to store many frames of image data which can be individually reviewed in turn using the cineloop control function. The actual number of stored frames in the image memory will vary according to the frame rate being used.

Sector width

The sector width, also referred to as the sector angle, is important in determining the frame rate at a given depth. The size of the sector width or angle can be reduced by the operator and is as illustrated in Figure 10.7.

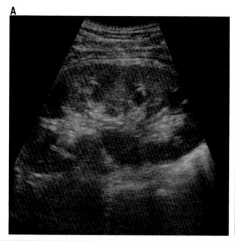
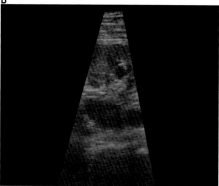

Fig. 10.7 • Illustrating sector width. a) B-mode image for a given depth, sector width and line density determines the frame rate. b) Image with a reduced sector width

B-mode images are made up of a number of adjacent scan lines; there can be many hundreds of scan lines used to form one image and the number of scan lines used is known as the line density. A sector width for a given depth and line density determines the frame rate and is seen in Figure 10.7a.

Reducing the sector width as seen in Figure 10.7b can bring about improvements to the overall frame rates and/or image resolution.

At a given depth, reducing the sector width means that fewer scan lines are required to form an image. This reduces the time needed to build up an image, resulting in higher frame rates. These high frame rates are required when imaging the heart, for example, and this technique of improving the overall frame rate is used especially when scanning the fetal heart in obstetrics.

Alternatively, reducing the sector width can bring about improvements to image resolution if the number of scan lines within this reduced sector is maintained, i.e. using thinner scan lines. This brings about no improvements to frame rates (they remain unchanged), but the increased line density increases the spatial resolution, namely lateral resolution.

The benefits of reducing the sector width are summarized in Table 10.1.

Zoom

If the region within the B-mode image is small or very deep the operator can use the zoom control to magnify an area of interest on the screen. The machine often allows the operator to adjust the size and position of the region of interest. There are two forms of zoom, read zoom and write zoom.

Read zoom simply magnifies the image, bringing about no improvements to the quality of the image. Using read zoom is similar to looking at news print very close up or using the digital zoom facility on modern digital cameras.

Real zoom, also known as write zoom, increases the ultrasound information content within the image, i.e. improves image resolution by increasing the scan line density and the number of pixels per square centimeter. The effect is similar to using a camera's optical zoom function.

On some machines it can be difficult to determine if the zoom facility is either read or write.

Dynamic range/log compression

Dynamic range refers to the way that the gray scale information is compressed into a usable range for display on the monitor. A broader or wide dynamic range yields more shades of gray, while a smaller or narrow dynamic range results in a more black and white appearance of the image. Figure 10.8 illustrates the effect that increasing the dynamic range has on the ultrasound image.

Since the range of signal amplitudes which are detected is so large, a decibel scale is used (dB). The dynamic range in decibels (dB) refers to the amount that the signal is compressed and expressed as the ratio of the largest to the smallest signal that can be visualized (white and black respectively).

For example, 60 dB represents a ratio of 1 000 000:1. The displayed dynamic range will affect the echo/gray scale assignment. A dynamic range of 40 dB (10 000:1 ratio) gives a highly contrasted image (see Fig. 10.8) that may be better for visualizing the walls of vessels, for example. Here, we are not interested in differentiating between a wide range of gray levels as blood appears black and vessel walls appear bright white. A dynamic range of 60 dB gives a softer image that may prove better for visualizing subtle differences within and between tissues, for example when scanning the liver as illustrated in Figure 10.8.

	BENEFIT	RESULT
Reducing the size of the sector width	– increases scan line density – more scan lines over the same area	– better detail – increased image resolution
	– fewer scan lines to process – increases frame rate	– increased temporal resolution

Table 10.1 Summarizing the benefits brought about by reducing the sector width

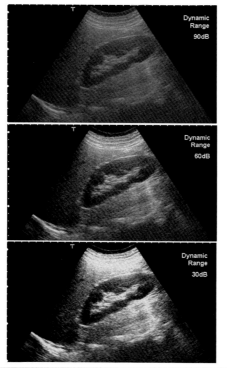

Increasing the dynamic range

Fig. 10.8 • Demonstrating the effect that increasing the dynamic range has on the overall ultrasound image

MEASUREMENTS

Measurement of key parameters within an ultrasound image is an essential part of interpreting ultrasound scans and aids with differentiating normal anatomy from pathology, monitoring fetal growth patterns, and are used to estimate due dates for delivery. Ultrasound machines are able to take a variety of measurements from frozen static B-mode images which include:

- linear
- circumference
- area
- volume.

SUMMARY

- A diagnostic ultrasound machine consists of many components which generate, process and display the received ultrasound signals
- Ultrasound machines have a large number of controls
- Each control influences image quality
- It is important for the operator to have an understanding of the function of each manual control in order to use them correctly
- Most ultrasound machines provide the operator with a range of preconfigured control settings known as presets
- A number of measurements can be taken with ultrasound equipment and form an essential part of interpreting ultrasound scans and differentiating normal anatomy from pathology

APPENDIX

EXERCISES TO IMPROVE YOUR UNDERSTANDING OF EQUIPMENT CONTROLS

The aim of these simple exercises is to become familiar with a number of B-mode imaging controls

PRESETS
- Select a type of examination (carotid, obstetrics, abdominal, cardiac, etc.)
- Make a note of the B-mode settings on the display and observe what alters as you change to different presets
- Select a preset and choose an appropriate transducer. Use either a test object/phantom or willing volunteer to obtain an ultrasound image

GAIN
- Notice what happens to the image if the gain control is altered

TGC
- Notice what happens to the image if the TGC slider controls are altered

DEPTH
- When you alter the depth control, do any other parameters displayed on the monitor change? (Pay close attention to the frame rate)

FOCUS
- What happens to the image when you move the focal zone up or down?
- What happens to the image if you select more than one focal zone?
- What other parameters displayed on the monitor change when you use more than one focal zone?

SECTOR WIDTH
- What parameters displayed on the monitor change when you reduce the sector width?

DYNAMIC RANGE
- What happens to the image when you change the dynamic range?

CINELOOP
- How many images can you review when you use the cineloop function?
- How is this related to the frame rate?

Reference

Thrush A, Hartshorne T 2005 Peripheral vascular ultrasound: how, why and when, Churchill Livingstone, Edinburgh, Fig. 2.11.

Physical principles of Doppler ultrasound

CONTENTS

LEARNING OBJECTIVES

1 Outline the basic principles of the Doppler effect and how it is applied in medical ultrasound.

2 Discuss the significance of the angle of the Doppler beam to obtain reliable Doppler signals.

3 Be aware of the relationship between blood flow velocity (V) and the Doppler shifted signals (F_d).

4 List the types of Doppler ultrasound instruments used in diagnostic ultrasound.

5 Describe continuous wave, color flow imaging, and spectral Doppler instruments.

6 Identify typical Doppler artifacts.

INTRODUCTION

This chapter provides the basic introduction to the physical principles and application of Doppler ultrasound in practice. The application of Doppler in ultrasound was first introduced in the 1980s and since then this technique has expanded in all specialist fields of practical ultrasonography.

A Doppler ultrasound is a non-invasive test that can be used to investigate movement and particularly evaluate blood flow in arteries and veins. It can also be used to provide information regarding the perfusion of blood flow in an organ or within an area of interest. A more recent application is the investigation of tissue wall motion when evaluating the heart (see Chapter 14 on New technology).

Doppler ultrasound can be used to diagnose many conditions, including:

- heart valve defects and congenital heart disease
- a blocked artery (arterial occlusion)
- narrowing (stenosis) of an artery
- blood clots (deep vein thrombosis)
- varicose veins (venous insufficiency)
- arteriovenous malformations
- movement of the cardiac wall.

THE DOPPLER PRINCIPLE

The Doppler principle is named after the mathematician and physicist Christian Johann Doppler who first described this effect in 1842 by studying light from stars. He demonstrated that the colored appearance of moving stars was caused by their motion relative to the earth. This relative motion resulted in either a red shift or blue shift in the light's frequency. This shift in observed frequencies of waves from moving sources is known as the Doppler effect and applies to sound waves as well as light waves.

The Doppler Effect

An everyday example which demonstrates the Doppler effect is highlighted in Figure 11.1. We are all aware that the pitch of an ambulance siren changes as we stop and listen to it as it drives by. The frequency that reaches you is higher as the ambulance approaches and lower as the ambulance passes by. This is a consequence of the Doppler effect.

What is happening is that the sound waves are compressed when an object producing sound is moving in the same direction as the waves. The listener (observer) therefore receives shorter wavelengths. However, when the source of sound has passed the listener, the waves are now moving in the opposite direction (away from the listener), the wavelength becomes longer and the listener therefore hears a change in frequency.

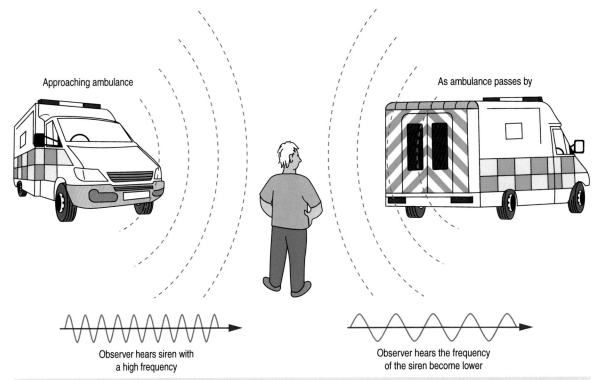

Approaching ambulance

As ambulance passes by

Observer hears siren with a high frequency

Observer hears the frequency of the siren become lower

Fig. 11.1 • The consequence of the Doppler effect on the relative emitted frequency of an ambulance siren as it drives by. The frequency of the approaching ambulance siren appears higher compared to the frequency of the siren as the ambulance passes by which appears lower

This Doppler effect is utilized in ultrasound applications to detect blood flow by analyzing the relative frequency shifts of the received echoes brought about by the movement of red blood cells.

THE DOPPLER EFFECT APPLIED TO DIAGNOSTIC ULTRASOUND

The Doppler effect in diagnostic imaging can be used to study blood flow, for example, and provides the operator with three pieces of information to determine:

- Presence or absence of flow
- Direction of blood flow
- Velocity of blood flow.

The transducer acts as both a transmitter and receiver of Doppler ultrasound. When using Doppler to investigate blood flow in the body, the returning backscattered echoes from blood are detected by the transducer. These backscattered signals (F_r) are then processed by the machine to detect any frequency shifts by comparing these signals to the transmitted Doppler signals (F_t). The frequency shift detected will depend on two factors, namely the magnitude and direction of blood flow (see Fig. 11.2).

Let us consider a simple arrangement as seen in Figure 11.3. The transducer transmits a Doppler signal with frequency F_t. The transmitted Doppler signal interrogates a blood vessel and the transducer receives the backscattered signals from the red blood cells within the vessel at a frequency

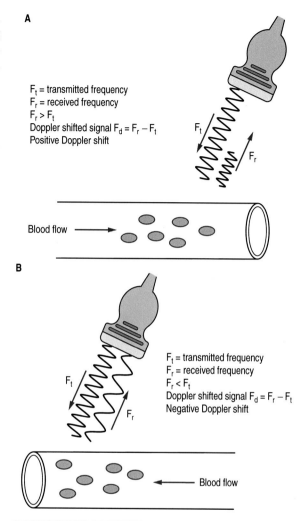

A

F_t = transmitted frequency
F_r = received frequency
$F_r > F_t$
Doppler shifted signal $F_d = F_r - F_t$
Positive Doppler shift

Blood flow

B

F_t = transmitted frequency
F_r = received frequency
$F_r < F_t$
Doppler shifted signal $F_d = F_r - F_t$
Negative Doppler shift

Blood flow

Fig. 11.3 • Demonstrating the resulting Doppler shifted signals for a) blood flow moving towards the transducer; b) blood flow moving away from the transducer

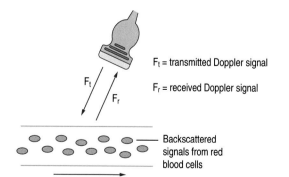

F_t = transmitted Doppler signal

F_r = received Doppler signal

Backscattered signals from red blood cells

Fig. 11.2 • An ultrasound transducer interrogating a blood vessel. Transmitting a Doppler signal with frequency F_t and receiving the backscattered signals from the red blood cells within the vessel at a frequency F_r

F_r. The Doppler frequency shift (F_d) can be calculated by subtracting the transmitted signal F_t from the received signal F_r.

Blood flow moving towards the transducer produces positive Doppler shifted signals and conversely blood flow moving away from the transducer produces negative Doppler shifted signals. Figure 11.3 illustrates the change in the received backscattered signals and the resulting Doppler shifts for blood moving towards and away from the transducer.

In Figure 11.3a the relative direction of the blood flow with respect to the Doppler beam is

75

towards the transducer. In this arrangement blood flow moving towards the transducer produces received signals (F_r) which have a higher frequency than the transmitted beam (F_t). The Doppler shifted signal (F_d) can be calculated by subtracting F_t from F_r and produces a positive Doppler shifted signal.

Conversely, Figure 11.3b illustrates blood flow which is moving away from the Doppler beam and the transducer. In this arrangement blood flow moving away from the transducer produces received signals (F_r) which have a lower frequency than the transmitted beam (F_t). This time the Doppler shifted frequencies ($F_r - F_t$) produces a negative Doppler shifted signal.

When there is no flow or movement detected then the transmitted frequency (F_t) is equal to the received frequency (F_r). Therefore $F_r = F_t$ and $F_d = F_r - F_t = 0$, resulting in no Doppler shifted signals.

It is important to appreciate that the amplitude of the backscattered echoes from blood is much weaker than those from soft tissue and organ interfaces which are used to build up our B-mode anatomical images. The amplitude of the backscattered signal from blood can be smaller by a factor of between 100 and 1000. Therefore highly sensitive and sophisticated hardware and processing software is required to ensure that these signals can be detected and processed.

THE DOPPLER EQUATION

The Doppler equation shows the mathematical relationship between the detected Doppler shifted signal (F_d) and the blood flow velocity (V):

$$F_d = \frac{2F_t V \cos\theta}{c}$$

where:

F_d = Doppler shifted signal

F_t = transmitted Doppler frequency

c = the propagation speed of ultrasound in soft tissue (1540 ms^{-1})

V = velocity of the moving blood

θ = the angle between the Doppler ultrasound beam and the direction of blood flow

The number 2 is a constant indicating that the Doppler beam must travel to the moving target and then back to the transducer.

Equation 1: The Doppler equation.

Relationship between Doppler Shifted Signal (F_d) and Blood Flow Velocity (V)

The Doppler equation (Equation 1) demonstrates that there is a relationship between the Doppler shifted signal (F_d) and the blood flow velocity (V). The Doppler shifted signal (F_d) is directly proportional to the blood flow velocity (V), which means greater flow velocities create larger Doppler shifted signals and conversely lower flow velocities generate smaller Doppler shifted signals. If we can detect and measure the value of F_d then the Doppler equation can be rearranged (see Equation 2) to calculate blood flow velocities (V) which can be processed and displayed.

$$V = \frac{F_d c}{2F_t \cos\theta}$$

Equation 2: Doppler equation rearranged to calculate blood flow velocities (V).

Significance of the Doppler Angle (θ)

Ultrasound machines are able to calculate Doppler shifted frequencies over a wide range of angles and it is important that an operator understands the significance of the angle of insonation (θ) between the Doppler beam and the direction of blood flow in vessels. Figure 11.4 graphically shows how the Doppler shifted signal changes as the Doppler beam angle changes.

When the Doppler beam is pointing towards the direction of blood flow a positive Doppler shifted signal is observed, but once the Doppler beam is pointed away from the direction of blood flow a negative Doppler shifted signal is seen. The smaller the angle between the Doppler beam and blood vessel, the larger the Doppler shifted signal. Very small signals are produced as the Doppler beam angle approaches a 90° angle.

Table 11.1 shows the relationship between the angle of the Doppler beam (θ) and the value of $\cos\theta$. The value of $\cos\theta$ varies with the angle from 0 to 1. When $\theta = 0°$, $\cos\theta = 1$ and when $\theta = 90°$, $\cos\theta = 0$.

For a constant flow velocity (V), the maximum value of $\cos\theta$ and therefore the highest value of the Doppler shifted signal (F_d) is at an angle of 0°. This corresponds to a Doppler beam which is

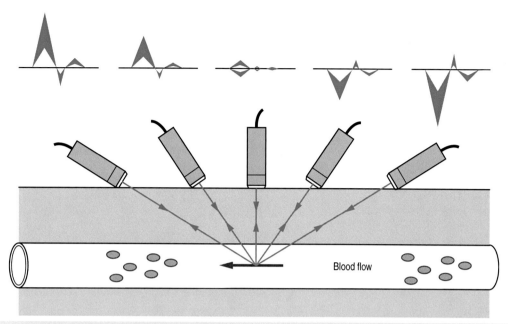

Fig. 11.4 • Graphically demonstrating the relationship between the Doppler shifted frequency with respect to the angle of the insonating Doppler beam

ANGLE θ	VALUE OF COSθ
0	1
30	0.87
45	0.71
60	0.5
75	0.26
90	0

Table 11.1 Variation of the value of cosθ over a range of angles of insonation. Maximum value of cosθ corresponds to a Doppler beam angle of 0°.

parallel with the vessel, which can rarely be achieved in practice.

Theoretically, when $θ = 90°$ this means the blood flow is perpendicular to the Doppler beam, $cosθ = 0$ and no Doppler shifted signals will register.

In practice, when taking measurements of blood flow, a Doppler beam angle of between 30 and 60° is important to ensure reliable Doppler shifted signals. Avoid using angles greater than

60° and remember no Doppler shifted signals are generated at 90°.

Greater flow velocities and smaller angles produce larger Doppler shifted frequencies, but not stronger Doppler shift signals.

Typical Doppler Shifted Signals for Blood Flow

Ultrasound machines transmit high-frequency sound waves which lie in the megahertz range, typically between 2 MHz and 20 MHz. Substituting typical physiological blood flow velocities into the Doppler equation gives Doppler shifted signals which lie within the audible range. That is, the range of frequencies that the human ear can hear. A healthy young human can usually hear from 20 cycles per second to around 20 000 cycles per second (20 Hz to 20 kHz).

Let us calculate a typical Doppler signal frequency for blood moving at 0.5 ms^{-1} which is illustrated in Figure 11.5. Transmitted frequency (F_t) is 4 MHz, $θ = 60°$ and c (the propagation speed of ultrasound) is assumed constant at 1540 ms^{-1}.

Using the Doppler equation (Equation 1) we calculate the Doppler shifted frequency to be

The Doppler equation

$$F_d = \frac{2F_t V\cos\theta}{c}$$

- Typical values
  - transmitted frequency   4 MHz
  - blood velocity   0.5 ms^{-1}
  - speed of sound   1540 ms^{-1}
  - θ 60°

  - Doppler shift frequency
  - F_d = 1299 cycles per second
  - F_d = 1300 Hz or 1.3 kHz
  - i.e. in audible range
  - simply can convert the Doppler shifted signal into an audible signal which can be heard through a loudspeaker

Fig. 11.5 • Illustrates the calculated Doppler shifted signal using the Doppler equation for blood flow moving at 50 cm/s for a Doppler beam operating at 4 MHz positioned with an insonation angle of 60°

1299 cycles per second, about 1300 Hz or abbreviated to 1.3 kHz.

These generated Doppler shifted signals can simply be converted into an audible signal which can be heard and monitored through a loudspeaker.

TYPES OF DOPPLER INSTRUMENTATION IN DIAGNOSTIC IMAGING

There are a number of types of Doppler instrumentation used in ultrasound which include:
- continuous wave Doppler
- color Doppler
- power Doppler
- spectral pulsed wave (PW) Doppler.

Doppler techniques applied to diagnostic ultrasound can be characterized as either being non-imaging or imaging. Non-imaging techniques typically use small or handheld units, and use continuous wave (CW) Doppler. The main purpose of these simple CW units is to either identify and/or monitor blood flow. Two examples of clinical examinations include fetal heart monitors in obstetrics and peripheral blood flow assessment in vascular practice.

Imaging Doppler techniques such as color and spectral PW Doppler are always used with B-mode imaging where the gray scale anatomical image is used to identify blood vessels and areas for blood flow evaluation. These techniques require more sophisticated processing than CW devices.

Continuous Wave Doppler Devices

Continuous wave (CW) Doppler devices are the simplest of Doppler instruments and typically consist of a handheld unit with an integrated speaker which is connected to a pencil probe transducer (Fig. 11.6).

The transducer consists of two piezoelectric elements: one element acts as a continuous transmitter (F_t) and the other acts as a continuous receiver (F_r).

These two elements are set at an angle to each other so that the transmit and reception beams overlap one another, as illustrated in Figure 11.7. This crossover region is known as the active or sensitive area and is where Doppler signals can only be detected. Doppler shift signals (F_d) are detected by comparing the transmitted and received signals: $F_d = F_r - F_t$.

The frequency and angle between the two elements within the transducer are determined by the clinical application.

For example, using CW Doppler in obstetrics for fetal heart monitoring requires a sufficiently low-frequency Doppler signal to be able to penetrate to the required depth; typically 4 MHz is used. The angle and therefore active crossover region between the two elements is also set to correspond to the required depth of integration.

Contrast this with the assessment of the peripheral circulation in the legs. Here the CW Doppler device is required to detect blood flow in vessels which lie very close to the skin surface. So here a higher Doppler transmit frequency can be used, typically 8 MHz, and the angle between

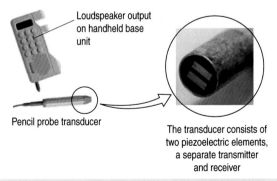

Loudspeaker output on handheld base unit

Pencil probe transducer

The transducer consists of two piezoelectric elements, a separate transmitter and receiver

Fig. 11.6 • A simple CW Doppler device illustrating the two piezoelectric elements at the tip of the pencil probe transducer: one acting as a continuous transmitter, the other acting as a continuous receiver

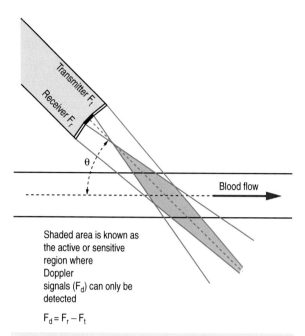

Shaded area is known as the active or sensitive region where Doppler signals (F_d) can only be detected

$$F_d = F_r - F_t$$

Fig. 11.7 • Elements within the transducer are set at a fixed angle. Doppler signals only detected where the transmitter and receiver beams overlap

CW DOPPLER DEVICES	
ADVANTAGES	**DISADVANTAGES**
Small	Cannot distinguish multiple vessels within crossover region
Cheap – simple design	Cannot measure velocity
Relatively easy to use and to search for a vessel	Unable to provide information about depth
Can display blood flow patterns	

Table 11.2 Comparative advantages and disadvantages of CW Doppler.

the two crystals within the probe is greater so that the crossover region corresponds to the required depth of only a couple of centimeters.

There are various CW Doppler devices available to detect blood flow. These range from simple inexpensive handheld Doppler units, where the Doppler signal is processed to provide an audible output, to more sophisticated devices which provide a visual display of the Doppler shifted blood flow patterns.

The main disadvantage of CW devices is that the transducer is sensitive to any blood flow within the crossover region. If more than one vessel is present in this crossover region then Doppler signals are obtained from more than one vessel at a time. Arteries and veins often lie adjacent to each other so in many cases CW devices will simultaneously detect arterial and venous flow signals. In addition, CW devices are unable to provide information on the depth from which the blood flow signals have returned and cannot measure blood flow velocity (V).

The advantages of CW Doppler devices are that they are small and cheap and are relatively easy to use with minimal training. Blood flow can be detected and monitored through a loudspeaker or blood flow patterns can be displayed graphically.

Table 11.2 summarizes the advantages and disadvantages of CW Doppler devices.

Doppler Imaging

There are three different types of Doppler imaging which will now be discussed:

  1 Color flow
  2 Power Doppler
  3 Spectral Doppler.

Color Flow Imaging

Color flow imaging was first introduced in the mid 1980s and since then has extended the role of ultrasound as a diagnostic tool. It can quickly and effectively enable the operator to identify the presence and direction of blood flow in vessels and can highlight gross circulation anomalies within the anatomical B-mode image.

It is probably the first Doppler technique that an operator will utilize to investigate blood flow. Color flow imaging is always used in conjunction with B-mode imaging and once it is activated the operator is presented with a region of interest known as the 'color box' and vertical 'color scale' bar which are superimposed onto the B-mode image, as illustrated in Figure 11.8.

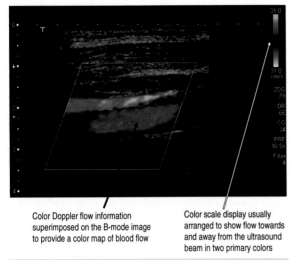

Color Doppler flow information superimposed on the B-mode image to provide a color map of blood flow

Color scale display usually arranged to show flow towards and away from the ultrasound beam in two primary colors

Fig. 11.8 • B-mode image with color flow information superimposed. Note that color flow information is only mapped into the color box region. Vertical color scale bar present on the right-hand side of the display

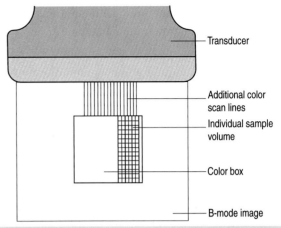

Fig. 11.9 • The color flow box is made up of hundreds of scan lines. Each scan line consists of hundreds of small sample volumes which individually detect the backscattered Doppler ultrasound signals

Unlike CW Doppler devices, where continuous Doppler beams are generated and transmitted by the two separate elements within the transducer, color flow imaging uses small groups of elements to transmit and receive the Doppler signals. The Doppler signals consist of a series of short bursts or pulses of ultrasound similar to those used in B-mode imaging. To form the color flow image, additional Doppler ultrasound pulses are generated by the transducer which is typically three to four times longer than those used for B-mode imaging. The transducer elements are rapidly switched between B-mode and color flow imaging to give an impression of a combined simultaneous image, and this is often known as duplex imaging, duplex meaning 'double'.

The position and size of this color box can be adjusted to the chosen area of interest by the operator to provide a visual color-coded display or map of blood flow.

The color box

The color image within the color box is made up of hundreds of scan lines which are each sub-divided into small sample volumes as illustrated in Figure 11.9. Typically, there are hundreds of sample volumes per scan line, amounting to thousands of sample volumes within the color box.

For each individual sample volume along each scan line, the average or mean Doppler shifted velocity is calculated. This mean Doppler shifted velocity, which can either be positive or negative, is assigned a color which is then mapped onto a color scale which consists of two primary colors. This is usually red for positive Doppler shifted signals (corresponding to blood flow traveling towards the transducer) and blue for negative Doppler shifted signals (corresponding to blood flow away from the transducer). This typical arrangement can be seen in Figure 11.8.

Once this directional information is processed, the sample volume is assigned a shade or hue depending on the calculated mean velocity.

The color flow information in the color box is made up by processing the information in each sample volume along each scan line in turn. In order to obtain a reliable estimation of the mean velocity in each sample volume, several (10 or more) pulse-echo sequences are required to produce each scan line of color flow information. This series of pulse-echo sequences is then repeated for the next adjacent scan line, and so on, as is the case for B-mode imaging.

A consequence of this multi pulse-echo technique is that it takes more time to collect and process the information required for color flow imaging than it does for standard B-mode imaging. As a result, color flow images tend to have lower frame rates than those used in B-mode.

Color scale

The color scale is represented as a vertical color bar and normally sits to the side of the B-mode image (see Fig. 11.8). Closer inspection of the color bar shows that it consists of two primary colors with each primary color subdivided into different shades or hues.

Just as in B-mode imaging, where returning echo amplitudes are assigned a varying level of gray to form the B-mode image (higher echo amplitudes are assigned brighter levels of gray and low amplitude echoes are assigned darker shades of gray), in color flow imaging similarly higher calculated mean flow velocities are assigned varying hues of red and blue. The higher the velocity, the brighter the shade or hue assigned.

Figure 11.10 illustrates a typical color scale bar used. As you can see, it consists of a vertical color bar which is split from the center into two primary colors. The center of a standard color bar scale represents zero or no flow. In this case, blood flow towards the transducer will be labeled red and blood flow away from the transducer is labeled

blue. However, in most equipment this color bar scale can be changed, if required, by the operator.

Significance of angle

With any Doppler technique, angle is important. The appearance of the color flow image is very much dependent on the operator to obtain a sufficient angle between the Doppler ultrasound beam and the vessel.

Curvilinear and phased array transducers have a radiating pattern of ultrasound beams that can produce complex color flow images, depending on the orientation of the arteries and veins with respect to the Doppler beam. This can be seen in Figure 11.11 which presents a color flow image of an umbilical cord.

Many peripheral vessels run parallel to the face of a linear transducer and perpendicular to the Doppler beam. If the angle of the Doppler beam with respect to the vessel is at 90°, little or no Doppler signal will be detected, as seen in Figure 11.12. When using a linear array transducer the operator is able to overcome this problem by electronically steering the Doppler beam. This is performed by altering the angle of the color box, as illustrated in Figure 11.13. The objective is to

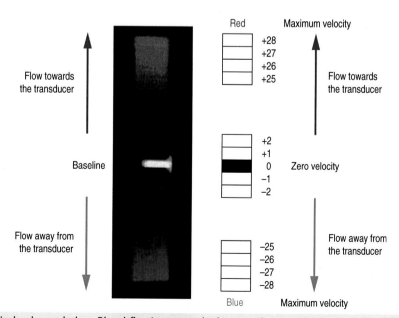

Fig. 11.10 • Typical color scale bar. Blood flowing towards the transducer is displayed as RED, blood flowing away from the transducer is BLUE. The brighter shades indicate higher velocities

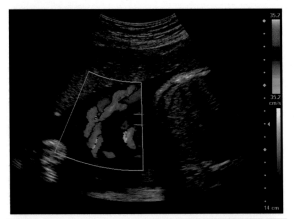

Fig. 11.11 • Color flow imaging of an umbilical cord highlighting the complex pattern of blood flow

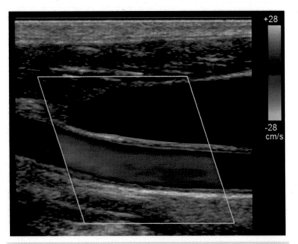

Fig. 11.13 • Color flow image of the common carotid artery with a steered color box to obtain sufficient angles for reliable Doppler signals

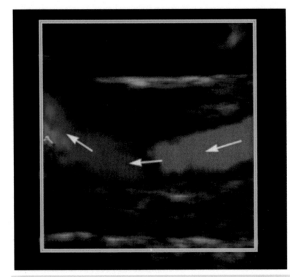

Fig. 11.12 • Color flow imaging demonstrating that no Doppler signal is registered when the vessel is at 90° with the Doppler beam

The color flow information is not built up continuously, as is the case with CW Doppler devices, but is formed from a series of Doppler ultrasound pulses which are transmitted at a given rate known as the sampling frequency.

In order to measure the many Doppler shifted frequencies present in typical blood flow patterns, thousands of pulses are sent along each scan line in turn. These sampled pulses are used to build up the Doppler shifted signal and in order to accurately build the Doppler shifted signal there must be an adequate number of samples per second.

Aliasing is the incorrect estimation of Doppler shifted signals due to undersampling which causes a false lower Doppler shifted frequency signal to appear in the sampled signal. Figure 11.14 shows

obtain a sufficiently small angle between the Doppler beam and blood vessel to provide reliable Doppler signals.

In practice, an experienced operator alters the scanning approach and steers the Doppler beam to obtain good angles between the Doppler beam and vessel to avoid unambiguous color flow images.

Aliasing

Aliasing occurs with all pulsed wave Doppler instruments because they employ a sampling method to build up the Doppler shifted signals.

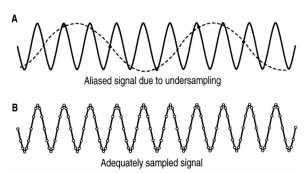

A Aliased signal due to undersampling

B Adequately sampled signal

Fig. 11.14 • a) Undersampled signal; b) adequately sampled signal

an undersampled signal and an adequately sampled signal of a simple sine wave.

In Figure 11.14a the undersampled signal appears to have a lower frequency than the actual signal – two cycles instead of ten cycles.

Increasing the sampling frequency as demonstrated in Figure 11.14b increases the number of data points acquired in a given time period. A rapid sampling frequency provides a better representation of the original signal than a slower sampling frequency.

The effect of aliasing can be seen when watching films where wagon wheels can appear to be going backwards instead of forwards due to the low frame rate of the film causing misinterpretation of the movement of the wheel spokes. The true velocity and correct direction of the wheel is only seen if the film's frame rate is rapid enough.

Significance of pulse repetition frequency

The frequency, i.e. sampling rate, at which these pulses can be sent is determined by the system's pulse repetition frequency (PRF) which can be adjusted through the color scale control button. Increasing the color scale increases the system's PRF and, conversely, reducing the color scale will reduce the system's PRF.

There is an upper limit to the system's PRF, i.e. color scale, which is restricted to the time the system has to wait to receive all the returning echoes along each scan line before sending another. This is linked to the maximum Doppler shifted signals (F_d) that can be detected. The maximum Doppler shifted signal F_d that can be measured is restricted, and is equal to half the pulse repetition frequency of the system, which is mathematically represented below:

$$F_d = \frac{PRF}{2}$$

This condition is known as the Nyquist limit. If the Nyquist limit is exceeded then aliasing will occur. When aliasing occurs, the displayed colors 'wrap around' the color scale bar and the colors change from the maximum color in one direction to the maximum in the opposite direction.

Figure 11.15a illustrates color aliasing which is caused when the color scale is set too low. The Doppler signals are undersampled at a PRF = 12.5 kHz which corresponds to a maximum color scale velocity of 13.9 cm/s. In this example, color flow changes from BLUE to RED are observed within the vessel. Increasing the color scale increases the PRF, from 12.5 kHz to 14 kHz, which is sufficient enough to eliminate aliasing within the image, as demonstrated in Figure 11.15b.

Significance of depth

A relationship exists between the maximum velocity of blood that can be detected and the maximum depth at which a vessel is investigated. As the depth

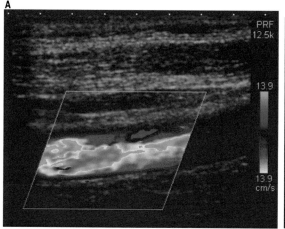
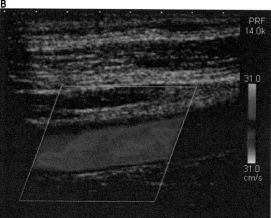

Fig. 11.15 • a) The color scale is set too low, resulting in aliasing of the color Doppler signal. The Doppler signals are undersampled at a PRF = 12.5 kHz. b) The color scale and PRF are increased to ensure that the Doppler signals are adequately sampled, resulting in the elimination of aliasing. This is achieved at a higher PRF of 14 kHz

of investigation increases, the journey time of the pulse to and from the reflector is increased; this in turn reduces the system's PRF. This reduction in the system's PRF reduces the maximum Doppler shifted signal (F_d) that can be displayed before aliasing occurs. The result is that the maximum Doppler shifted signals (F_d) which can be measured decrease with depth.

Advantages and limitations of color flow imaging

Advantages

- Gives an overall view of flow within a region
- Indicates flow direction
- Identifies areas of turbulent flow velocities and anomalies
- Indicates absence of flow in occluded vessels.

Limitations include

- Flow information limited to mean velocity
- Poor temporal resolution – frame rate can be low when scanning deep
- Subject to aliasing
- Angle dependent.

Power Doppler

Power Doppler is also referred to as energy Doppler, amplitude Doppler and Doppler angiography. It is a color flow imaging technique that maps the magnitude, i.e. power, of the backscattered Doppler signal rather than the Doppler shifted flow velocities. The instantaneous signal strength contained in the Doppler signal is calculated and superimposed onto the B-mode image as illustrated in Figure 11.16. Its effect is to provide a map of areas of perfusion, by displaying the amplitude of red blood cells in an area.

Power Doppler does not display the relative velocity and direction of blood flow as is the case with color flow imaging. Power Doppler uses a single color scale and maps increasing signal strengths to increased luminosity. It is often used in conjunction with frame averaging to increase sensitivity to low flows and velocities.

Power Doppler has several advantages over color flow imaging which include:

- being more sensitive to flow and detecting low flows. The display of backscattered power is independent of angle

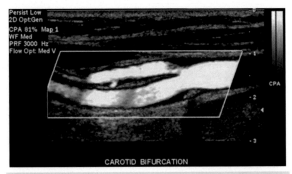

Fig. 11.16 • Power Doppler image of the carotid bifurcation

- not being subject to aliasing as it does not use a sampling technique
- providing better edge detection, e.g. around arterial plaques.

But it has the disadvantages of:

- displaying no direction of flow velocity information
- being subject to very poor temporal resolution – a high degree of frame averaging is used
- being extremely sensitive to motion – which means that the transducer needs to be kept still to give good images.

Spectral or Pulse Wave Doppler

Spectral Doppler, also referred to as pulsed wave (PW) Doppler, is combined with B-mode and color flow imaging techniques and allows for the assessment and evaluation of the blood flow over a very small region known as the sample volume. This technique is known as range gating.

When spectral Doppler is initially instigated, a single Doppler beam axis is superimposed onto the B-mode and color flow image as illustrated in Figure 11.17. The size and position of the sample volume can be adjusted anywhere along the axis of the Doppler beam and this information is displayed on the monitor. The position of the sample volume determines where along the Doppler beam blood flow velocities are to be investigated. The size of the sample volume determines how much of the vessel is examined. For arterial examinations, the sample volume is positioned in the

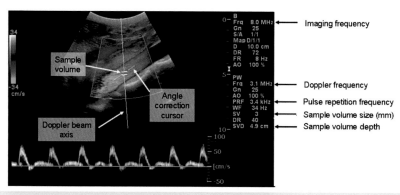

Fig. 11.17 • Illustration of the on-screen components when spectral Doppler is activated. Highlighting the Doppler beam axis, the sample volume, and angle correction cursor. The size and position of the sample volume is always displayed on screen

center of the vessel, and the size of the sample volume is set to be approximately one half to one third of the diameter of the vessel.

When the sample volume has been correctly positioned over a point of interest then the spectral Doppler display is activated to provide blood flow velocity information.

The Doppler beam itself can be maneuvered over the B-mode image and follows the path of the B-mode imaging scan lines for a sector array transducer, as depicted in Figure 11.17. When linear array transducers are used, the Doppler beam can be steered, which enables the operator to achieve the necessary angle between the Doppler beam and blood vessel under investigation. An example of this is shown in Figure 11.18.

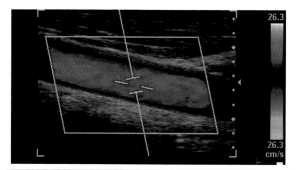

Fig. 11.18 • An example of a linear array transducer electronically steering both the color and spectral Doppler beams to obtain a sufficient angle between the Doppler beam and blood vessel for reliable Doppler assessment

The angle correction cursor which is located at the center of the sample volume is used to estimate the angle of insonation between vessel and Doppler beam and should be adjusted to align with the direction of blood flow in the vessel to calculate absolute flow velocities from the detected Doppler shifted signals.

By angle correcting, the operator provides the ultrasound system with the actual value of θ in the Doppler equation. Once θ is known, the Doppler equation can be used to calculate actual blood flow velocities. Accurate and reliable spectral Doppler flow velocities are achieved for angles of θ, between the Doppler beam and the direction of blood flow, which are no greater than 60°.

Color flow imaging which maps blood flow over a much larger area is used in conjunction with spectral Doppler, highlighting areas of disturbed or turbulent blood flow for spectral Doppler assessment.

Spectral Doppler, combined with real-time B-mode and color flow imaging, is known as triplex imaging. When triplex imaging is used by the operator, data collecting and processing is shared between all three modes. This reduces the overall imaging frame rate and Doppler sampling frequency, which in turn restricts the range over which blood flow velocities can be measured.

Optimum spectral Doppler assessments are achieved when B-mode and color flow imaging modes are temporarily frozen which allows more time to be employed for rapid spectral Doppler processing.

Generation of spectral PW Doppler signals

Spectral Doppler is similar to color flow imaging in the way that it utilizes a sampling technique to build up the spectral Doppler shifted signals. As is the case for B-mode imaging, a small group of elements within the transducer acts as both a transmitter and receiver of Doppler ultrasound, transmitting regular short bursts of spectral Doppler signals from which received Doppler shifted signals are processed. However, spectral Doppler only sends out one beam, unlike color Doppler which requires many adjacent beams to form the color flow image. The pulses generated for spectral Doppler differ from those used for B-mode imaging and tend to be longer, typically 6–10 cycles in length.

Processing and displaying the PW Doppler signal

Spectral Doppler provides more detailed information of blood flow than color flow imaging and is able to map the variation and distribution of blood flow velocities over the cardiac cycle. The spectral Doppler signal contains all this information.

Doppler signals are processed using spectral analysis to provide a more meaningful and useful way to represent the Doppler velocity information visually. Spectral analysis breaks down the Doppler signals received within the sample volume into its range of frequency components, which are translated into a range of flow velocities. The process of spectral analysis can be thought of as being similar to using a prism to split visible light into its separate components, i.e. its color spectrum, as seen in Figure 11.19.

Figure 11.20 shows a typical spectral analysis trace for a femoral artery, with time along the

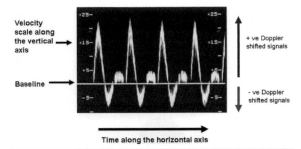

Fig. 11.20 • Spectral waveform of a femoral artery displaying time along the horizontal axis and flow velocities along the vertical axis

horizontal axis and flow velocities (calculated from the Doppler shifted signals) along the vertical axis. The vertical axis is divided into two so that both positive and negative Doppler shifted signals can be displayed. The baseline relates to zero flow. Both the velocity scale and baseline can be adjusted by the operator to ensure that spectral waveforms are optimally displayed.

The third axis of the spectral trace corresponds to the backscattered power of the Doppler shifted signal at each velocity. This is simply displayed as brightness which is illustrated in Figure 11.21.

Spectral analysis is performed by the ultrasound machine's on-board computer using a mathematical technique known as a fast Fourier transform (FFT) and produces between 100–200 lines of processed data every second. PW Doppler systems are able to process information fast enough to produce real-time spectral Doppler waveforms and, as a consequence of this, rapid processing is said to have good temporal resolution.

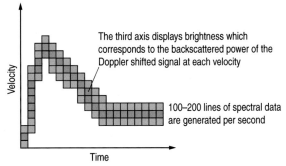

Fig. 11.21 • A spectral analysis trace displaying the variation of velocities over the cardiac cycle. The brightness corresponds to the backscattered power of the Doppler shifted signal at each velocity

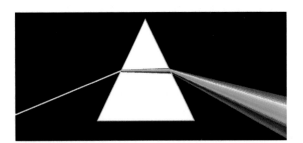

Fig. 11.19 • A prism splitting light into its individual components is similar to the process employed by spectral analysis

Aliasing

Because spectral Doppler uses a sampling technique to interrogate and build up information about the blood flow velocities, it is subject to aliasing. As discussed under Color Flow Imaging, aliasing is governed by the system's Doppler PRF which can be adjusted through the spectral Doppler 'scale' control. The maximum velocity that can be measured is directly proportional to half the value of the PRF. The higher the pulse repetition frequency of the Doppler pulses, the higher the Doppler shifted velocity that can be measured. The PRF is also linked to the position (i.e. the depth) of the sample volume. The deeper the sample volume is placed within the B-mode image, the lower the value of the PRF due to time constraints, i.e. the system has to wait longer to receive the reflected Doppler pulses from a sample volume which is placed deep within the image rather than one which is positioned close to the transducer. The relationship between PRF, the maximum measurable velocity, and the depth of the sample volume are summarized in Table 11.3.

The effects of aliasing are demonstrated in Figure 11.22 and cannot always be eliminated, as it is not always possible to have the PRF significantly higher than the Doppler shifted signal. However, these effects can be minimized by adjusting the following controls:

- Increase vertical spectral velocity scale which in turn increases the system's PRF
- Offset zero baseline on PW spectrum which is only possible if the flow is significantly in one direction

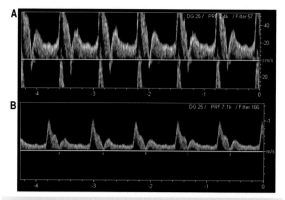

Fig. 11.22 • Example of aliasing and correction of the aliasing. a) Waveforms with aliasing wrap around the velocity scale resulting in the peaks being displayed below the baseline. b) Aliasing avoided with the same spectral waveform achieved by increasing the pulse repetition frequency, i.e. increasing the velocity scale

- Reduce transmitted frequency (F_t) as the Doppler equation shows that the Doppler shifted frequency (F_d) is proportional to F_t so lower F_t will lower the value of F_d
- Reduce the angle (θ) between the Doppler beam and vessel.

Advantages and disadvantages of spectral Doppler

Advantages

- Examines flow at one site
- Good temporal resolution – gives detailed analysis of distribution of blood flow velocities over the cardiac cycle
- Can make calculations of flow velocities.

ACTION		CONSEQUENCE
As PRF increases	Maximum measurable velocity increases	
As PRF decreases	Maximum measurable velocity decreases	
As the depth of sample volume increases	PRF decreases	Maximum measurable velocity decreases
As the depth of sample volume decreases	PRF increases	Maximum measurable velocity increases

Table 11.3 Demonstrating the relationship between PRF, maximum measurable velocity, and depth of sample volume.

Disadvantages

- Uses a sampling technique and therefore is subject to aliasing
- Limit on maximum velocity that can be measured – governed by PRF
- Angle dependent.

Table 11.4 summarizes and compares these three Doppler modes.

DOPPLER ARTIFACTS

Aliasing

Aliasing is the most common Doppler artifact and occurs with all pulsed wave Doppler instruments because they employ a sampling method to build up the Doppler shifted signals. Aliasing is the incorrect estimation of Doppler shifted signals due to undersampling. When aliasing occurs, the displayed Doppler shifted signals 'wrap around' the Doppler velocity scale and the Doppler shifted signals change from the maximum velocity in one direction to the maximum in the opposite direction. Figures 11.15 and 11.22 demonstrate the effects of aliasing upon the color and spectral Doppler imaging displays.

Doppler Mirror Image

This type of artifact can be seen in both spectral Doppler and color flow imaging.

This mirror artifact can be seen in spectral Doppler traces where there is electronic duplication of spectral information being displayed below the zero baseline, as seen in Figure 11.23. It commonly results from the Doppler receiver gain being set too high.

Color images can also produce mirror artifacts and can normally be seen where a vessel lies above a strong reflecting surface. Figure 11.24 shows a mirror image of the subclavian artery produced by multiple reflections from the pleura above the lung, where there is a soft-tissue/air boundary present, causing strong reflections.

DOPPLER FLOW IMAGING MODE	MAIN ADVANTAGES AND DISADVANTAGES
Color flow imaging	- Gives an overall view of flow within a region - Identifies turbulent flow velocities - Flow information limited to mean velocity - Poor temporal resolution – frame rate can be low when scanning deep - Subject to aliasing - Angle dependent
Power Doppler	- Sensitive to low flows - No directional information - Very poor temporal resolution – susceptible to transducer movement - Not angle dependent
Spectral Doppler	- Examines flow at one site - Good temporal resolution – gives detailed analysis of distribution of blood flow velocities over the cardiac cycle - Can make calculations of flow velocities - Subject to aliasing - Limit on maximum velocity that can be measured – governed by PRF - Angle dependent

Table 11.4 Comparison and summary of Doppler flow imaging modes.

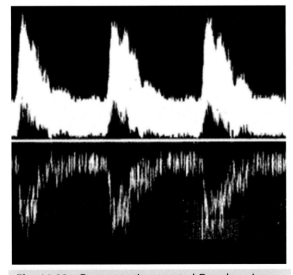

Fig. 11.23 • Demonstrating spectral Doppler mirror artifact due to the receiver gain being set too high

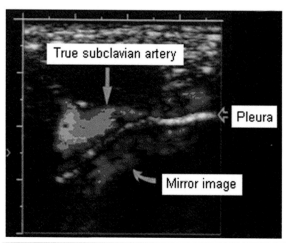

Fig. 11.24 • Color image of the subclavian artery with a mirror image below the pleura

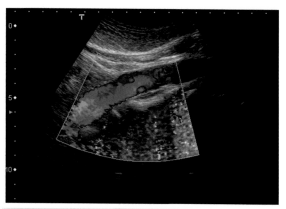

Fig. 11.25 • Demonstrating flashes of color seen within the image brought about by rapid movements of either the transducer or tissues by respiration

Flash artifact

Both color flow and power Doppler imaging use filters to suppress signals arising from stationary or near stationary tissue. However, large movements of tissues brought about by heavy respiration or rapid transducer movement, for example, can cause significant flashes of color across large areas within the color flow image. Some machines have motion suppression algorithms to reduce this flash artifact. This is illustrated in Figure 11.25.

SUMMARY

- The Doppler effect can be applied in diagnostic ultrasound to detect the movement of internal structures and the motion of blood flow
- There is a range of Doppler instruments available, from simple handheld CW devices to more complicated and sophisticated Doppler imaging machines
- Doppler imaging instruments make use of the Doppler effect to process information which can display the motion, direction, and velocity of blood flow
- Doppler signals are subject to angle dependence
- Color flow imaging and spectral Doppler use a sampling technique to build up the Doppler signals and as a consequence of this are subject to aliasing
- Artifacts can occur with Doppler ultrasound instruments and include aliasing, mirroring, and flash artifact

Ultrasound safety

LEARNING OBJECTIVES

1 Outline the parameters used to describe the strength of an ultrasound beam.

2 Discuss the significance of different operating modes and their potential risk of producing biological effects.

3 Be aware of current diagnostic ultrasound output limits.

4 Describe the thermal and non-thermal physical mechanisms that can cause biological effects.

5 Explain the thermal index (TI) and mechanical index (MI) and understand the significance of these in relation to causing a potential biological hazard.

6 Be aware of the general guidelines offered by ultrasound organizations and societies.

7 Discuss the influence of the machine controls.

8 Outline the ways to limit exposure by adopting the ALARA principle.

9 Have a basic appreciation of epidemiological evidence.

INTRODUCTION

There has been a considerable and rapid growth in the use of ultrasound as a diagnostic imaging tool over the past 50 years since it was first used to image the unborn fetus. This rapid growth has resulted in millions of people worldwide being scanned every year. Changes and advances in technology are leading to increasing power levels being used to obtain diagnostic information. The interaction of ultrasound with biological tissue can result in effects which may cause heating, interfere with the normal functioning of cells, and cause structural damage. The potential damaging nature of ultrasound leads to concern over its safety. All operators therefore need to have an understanding of the safety implications in order to practice safely.

WHY ARE WE INTERESTED?

Ultrasound is a mechanical form of energy which interacts with the biological tissue through which it travels. Millions of women have their pregnancy routinely scanned with ultrasound and any adverse effects are more likely to damage the rapidly developing cells found in embryo, fetus, and neonate.

New research is continually being carried out, but variable parameters of ultrasound exposure and mechanisms of interaction with tissue lead to problems in determining when safe levels are being breached.

Important Parameters

Amplitude, power, and intensity are parameters used to describe the strength of an ultrasound beam.

Amplitude

Amplitude is a measure of a wave's magnitude of oscillation, that is, the magnitude of the maximum disturbance in the medium, and in ultrasound often refers to the maximum variation (see Fig. 12.1). Amplitude is measured in units of pressure: MPa (megapascals).

Power (P)

Power in ultrasound describes the rate at which energy is generated and transferred by the acoustic wave per unit of time. Power is measured in watts (W) and milliwatts (mW), one milliwatt being one thousandth of a watt. Power is proportional to the square of the amplitude, i.e. if the power is doubled then the amplitude is quadrupled.

Intensity (I)

Intensity is the rate at which energy passes through the unit area and is an important quantity when discussing bioeffects and safety.

The average intensity is equal to the power of an ultrasound beam, normally expressed in mW, divided by the cross-sectional area of the beam, expressed in cm^2. Units of intensity for diagnostic ultrasound are typically expressed in $mWcm^{-2}$.

From the equation in Figure 12.2 we can identify that the intensity of an ultrasound beam is directly proportional to its power, i.e. if beam power increases, then intensity increases and, conversely, if beam power decreases, the intensity decreases.

In addition, we can see that intensity is also inversely proportional to the beam area, i.e. if the beam area decreases, then the beam intensity increases and, conversely, if the beam area increases, the beam intensity decreases.

The maximum intensity along an ultrasound beam lies at the focus (the narrowest part of the beam)

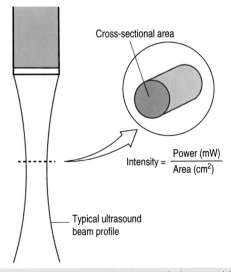

Cross-sectional area

$$\text{Intensity} = \frac{\text{Power (mW)}}{\text{Area (cm}^2)}$$

Typical ultrasound beam profile

Fig. 12.2 • Diagram showing a typical ultrasound beam profile and a cross-sectional area. Cross-sectional area varies with depth and is smallest at the focus where the intensity is the highest

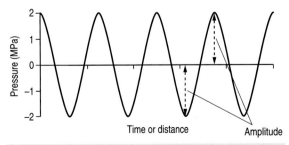

Time or distance

Amplitude

Fig. 12.1 • Demonstrating the varying pressure amplitude of an oscillating acoustic wave

where all the power is concentrated into a small cross-sectional area.

The intensity within an ultrasound beam also varies from point to point across the beam (spatial considerations), as demonstrated in Figure 12.3. Two values of intensity can de defined:

- Spatial peak intensity (I_{SP}) – is the highest intensity and is found at the center of the beam
- Spatial average intensity (I_{SA}) – is the average intensity across the beam and takes account of the variation across the width of the beam.

Because of the pulsed nature of ultrasound, the intensity of the ultrasound beam also varies over time (temporal considerations). Figure 12.4 shows the relevant times for three intensities:

- Temporal peak intensity (I_{TP}) – is the highest intensity found in a pulse and is not averaged over time

- Pulse average intensity (I_{PA}) – is the intensity averaged over the pulse duration. Lies in between I_{TP} and I_{TA}
- Temporal average intensity (I_{TA}) – takes account of the 'dead' time between pulses and is averaged over the pulse repetition period (PRP). It is the lowest value.

These spatial and temporal variations within the ultrasound beam result in the fact that there are a number of ways of defining intensity, as detailed below:

Highest intensity

I_{SPTP} – Spatial peak-temporal peak (SPTP)

I_{SATP} – Spatial average-temporal peak (SATP)

I_{SPPA} – Spatial peak-pulse average (SPPA)

I_{SAPA} – Spatial average-pulse average (SAPA)

I_{SPTA} – Spatial peak-temporal average (SPTA)

Lowest intensity

I_{SATA} – Spatial average-temporal average (SATA)

I_{SPTA} is the measure most associated with temperature rises.

OPERATING MODES AND THEIR POTENTIAL RISK

For any operating mode there is a large variation of output powers and intensities. The output data for all modern day ultrasound machines can be sourced from the operator's manual.

Exposures used in Doppler modes such as spectral pulsed Doppler and color flow imaging are higher than for B and M modes.

B modes

Uses the lowest output power and intensities and is generally considered safe in all applications.

Pulsed Doppler

The longer pulses, higher powers, and pulse repetition rates typically used in pulsed Doppler result in higher average intensities compared to B-mode imaging and therefore there is an increased potential of producing a biological effect, particularly from ultrasound-induced heating.

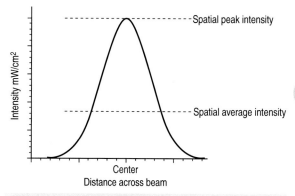

Fig. 12.3 • Demonstrating the variation of intensity across an ultrasound beam. The spatial intensity across the beam is at its highest at the center, tailing off towards the edges

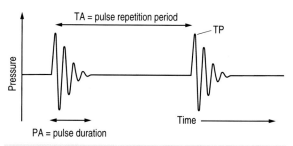

Fig. 12.4 • Demonstrating the three time-dependent intensities

93

Dwell time, i.e. the length of time that the ultrasound beam is fixed on a specific tissue area, is an important factor when considering the potential for heating. This is particularly relevant for spectral pulsed Doppler where the beam is held in a fixed position during an investigation; this leads to a further increase in temporal average intensity and therefore increased risk of causing a temperature rise.

Color Flow Mapping and Power Doppler Imaging Modes

These modes involve some beam scanning, and so generally have a heating potential that is somewhere between that of B-mode and that of spectral pulsed Doppler.

Table 12.1 summarizes data collected from a survey conducted by Henderson in 1997. Here you can see that the highest intensities are produced when using pulsed Doppler modes.

WHO REGULATES ULTRASOUND ACOUSTIC OUTPUT LIMITS?

Surprisingly enough, these are not regulated by a medical body. Regulations governing the output of diagnostic ultrasound have been largely set by the USA's Food and Drug Administration (FDA). In 1991 the FDA relaxed its regulations and increased the permissible acoustic output and intensity levels used to scan early pregnancy to almost eight times over the level that had been previously allowed (from 94 to 720 mWcm^{-2}). Table 12.2 shows these changes in acoustic output levels in relation to the range of diagnostic areas.

However, for the manufacturers to utilize these increased output levels and higher intensities, it was agreed that their equipment should provide an on-screen display relating to the acoustic output. Its purpose is to inform the user of the potential risk for an examination to produce a biological effect. This shifted the onus of safety to the end user who is now responsible for making a risk/benefit assessment. This requires the ultrasound user to understand the potential for biological effects and practice to ensure exposure times are kept to a minimum.

OUTPUT DISPLAY STANDARDS

In 1992, the American Institute of Ultrasound in Medicine (AIUM) and the National Electrical Manufacturers Association (NEMA) defined a set of output display standards (ODS). For each ultrasound examination, a real-time on-screen display indicates the risk of producing biological effects. ODS is based on two indices which give two main measures of output:

- TI = Thermal effects (related to average intensity)
- MI = Cavitation – non-thermal (related to peak pressure).

This enables users to be aware of output levels during scanning.

These increases in output levels have also driven some of the improvements and developments in diagnostic ultrasound that we mentioned earlier, to the extent that modern ultrasound equipment is capable of producing measurable biological effects in tissues (Barnett 1998, Barnett & Kossoff 1992).

BIOLOGICAL EFFECTS OF ULTRASOUND

Physical Mechanisms

Clinically we know ultrasound energy can be utilized in lithotripsy by using a focused, high-intensity acoustic pulse to destroy a kidney stone.

OPERATING MODE	POWER	MEAN I$_{SPTA}$ (mWcm^{-2})	POTENTIAL RISK
Pulsed Doppler	Highest	1700	Highest risk for possible heating
Color Doppler		450	Risk of heating with small color boxes
B mode	Lowest	200	Considered safe

Table 12.1 Values of the UK survey of equipment in clinical use (from Henderson et al 1997).

APPLICATION	BEFORE 1991 (PRE ODS) INTENSITY LIMIT (I_{SPTA}) ($mWcm^{-2}$)	AFTER 1991 WITH ODS INTENSITY LIMIT (I_{SPTA}) ($mWcm^{-2}$)
Fetal, neonatal imaging	94	720
Cardiac	430	720
Peripheral vascular	720	720
Ophthalmology	17	50

Table 12.2 Shows the changes to maximum allowable output exposure following the changes stipulated by the US FDA. ODS; output display standards.

These devices use energies much higher than those utilized in diagnostic ultrasound, however it can be easily demonstrated that there is potential for destruction.

There are two distinct mechanisms that can cause biological effects on tissue when exposed to ultrasound. These are:

- Thermal (heating)
- Non-thermal effects (cavitation).

Thermal effects

As the ultrasound beam travels through tissue, some of its energy is lost through absorption. This absorbed energy is converted into heat which in turn produces a temperature rise. In most soft tissues, the rate at which energy is absorbed depends on the:

- attenuation coefficient of the tissue
- operating frequency
- power/intensity of the ultrasound beam
- length of operating time (exposure time).

The thermal effect is highest in tissues with a high absorption coefficient such as bone, and is low where there is little absorption such as amniotic fluid (water).

The potential of any temperature rise also depends on the thermal characteristics of the tissue to dissipate this heat to surrounding areas, the ultrasound intensity, and the length of time for which the tissue volume is scanned.

Frequency is another factor and the higher the operating frequency, the higher the absorption and potential to cause heat. This is particularly significant when using endocavity probes which use higher frequencies to improve image quality.

The ultrasound intensity varies along the ultrasound beam and is greatest at the focus where the beam is at its narrowest. The intensity can be changed by other operator controls such as power output, scan depth, and mode of operation, i.e. using color and Doppler modes.

Heat can also be produced at the transducer surface which can be directly transferred to the tissue it is in contact with. This can be particularly significant when using transvaginal probes to investigate a pregnancy during the first eight weeks postconception.

The World Federation for Ultrasound in Medicine and Biology (WFUMB; Barnett 1998), following a review of the literature on the effects of temperature elevation on animal fetuses, concluded that a temperature rise of no more than 1.5°C may be used clinically without reservation, however, exposures that elevate embryonic and fetal temperatures higher than 4°C for 5 minutes or more should be considered as potentially hazardous.

Thermal index (TI)

The thermal index (TI) as defined by AIUM/NEMA is the ratio of the acoustic power produced by the transducer (W) to the power required to raise the temperature in tissue by 1°C (W_{deg}). This is mathematically expressed in Equation 1:

$$TI = \frac{W}{W_{deg}}$$

Equation 1: Formula for thermal index.

(Derated values compensate for attenuation by soft tissue. Acoustic output measurements are usually performed in a water tank. To take into account the attenuation by soft tissue in practice, these values are adjusted, i.e. 'derated', using a value of attenuation of 0.3 dB/cm/MHz.)

A thermal index of 1 indicates the acoustic power achieving a temperature increase of 1°C. A thermal index of 2 has doubled power but would not necessarily indicate a peak temperature rise of 2°C. The algorithms in the machine which calculate TI are based on many assumptions and take into account a worst case scenario such as low levels of beam attenuation, a stationary beam, and fairly long exposure times.

There are several classifications of thermal indices:

- TIS – this is the thermal index applied when you are scanning through a soft-tissue structure and will probably be the one you most often encounter
- TIB – this is the thermal index which applies if bone is at or near the focus of the transducer. Remember, because of its high acoustic absorption, there is an increased potential for heating which will be reflected in the values of TI displayed. TIB is most appropriate for fetal ultrasound during the second or third trimester pregnancy scan where the highest temperature increase would be expected occurring at the soft tissue/bone interface.
- TIC – this is the thermal index applied when scanning cranial bone. Here, the bone is at or very near the skin surface.

Cavitation effects

Ultrasound produces an oscillating pressure wave which propagates through tissues. This propagating pressure wave can cause micro-bubbles within tissues to form, grow, oscillate in size and, at sufficiently high intensities and pressure, cause these bubbles to collapse. Small laboratory mammalian experiments have demonstrated this effect in lung and intestine, where small gas bubbles can be present. The most important sources of cavitation are those introduced during contrast studies.

Above diagnostic output levels, cavitation plays an important role in the destruction of kidney stones in shock wave lithotripsy.

There are two forms of cavitation:

- Stable (also known as non-inertial)
- Unstable (also known as transient or inertial).

Stable cavitation (non-inertial)

This form of cavitation is the process where small micro-bubbles in a medium are forced to oscillate in the presence of the ultrasound. The cavitation bubbles go through phases of expansion and contraction as they oscillate with the varying ultrasound pressure wave. Generally, this form of stable cavitation is regarded as being safe. Figure 12.5 graphically demonstrates the phases of bubble compression and contraction through the varying ultrasound pressure wave.

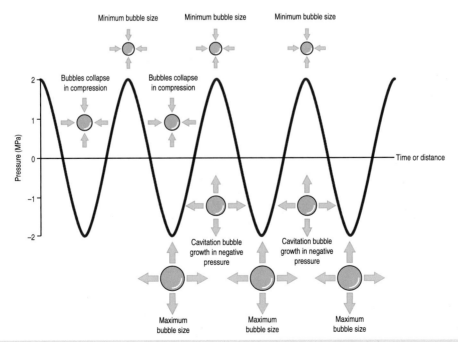

Fig. 12.5 • Demonstrating the phases of bubble compression and expansion through the varying ultrasound pressure wave. Size of bubble is smallest when compressed during the peak positive pressure and is largest during the peak negative or rarefaction pressure

Unstable cavitation (transient or inertial)

This type of cavitation has the greatest potential to damage tissue. Here, the intensity of the ultrasound field is high enough to cause the oscillations of the micro-bubbles to become so great that the bubbles collapse, generating high pressures and temperatures to the localized area, increasing the potential to cause biological damage. This effect has been demonstrated in small mammalian animal experiments causing lung capillary bleeding at pressure thresholds of 1 MPa which is well within the diagnostic range. Although this process has been reported in mammalian experiments, it has not been observed in humans. However, knowledge that there is a potential risk and hazard for biological damage due to this form of destructive cavitation is especially pertinent in early pregnancy where the tissues are more susceptible to this form of damage.

The use of contrast agents in the form of stabilized gas bubbles increases the probability of cavitation.

Mechanical index (MI)

The mechanical index (MI) is related to the likelihood of cavitation being produced and is defined as the peak rarefactional pressure (Pr) (negative pressure) divided by the square root of the ultrasound frequency:

$$MI = \frac{\text{Peak negative pressure (Pr) (Megapascals)}}{\sqrt{\text{Frequency}} \quad \text{(MHz)}}$$

Equation 2: Formula for calculating mechanical index.

The value of Pr (negative pressure) is significant here and from Equation 2 we can see that the value of MI is directly proportional to Pr. This means if Pr doubles then MI doubles and, conversely, if Pr is halved then MI is halved. Also we can see that frequency is inversely related to MI which means as frequency increases the value of MI actually decreases.

The FDA ultrasound regulations allow a mechanical index of up to 1.9 to be used for all applications except ophthalmic (maximum 0.23). The used range varies from 0.05 to 1.9.

It is stipulated that the values of the TI and MI must be displayed if the ultrasound system is capable of exceeding an index of 1.

The TI and MI are not absolute values but represent a rough approximation of the risk of creating certain biological effects. The higher the index value, the higher the potential of a biological effect.

PRUDENT USE – THE ALARA PRINCIPLE

Changes in power output and increased use of Doppler ultrasound, together with a change in regulations governing output, mean that the onus of safety is placed on the operator. As a consequence, every measure should be taken to ensure safe practice.

All ultrasound users should regularly check both thermal and mechanical indices while scanning and should adjust the machine controls to keep them as low as reasonably possible without compromising the diagnostic value of the examination. Where low values cannot be achieved, examination times should be kept as short as possible.

The ALARA ('As Low As Reasonably Achievable') principle should be applied and maintained. Minimize any possible risks by minimizing exposure times and exposure intensity.

GENERAL GUIDELINES

There are many safety guidelines issued by several national and international ultrasound societies and organizations to assist all those who use diagnostic ultrasound so that they are able to make informed decisions about ultrasound safety. These guidelines are based on the best scientific information available at the time.

A list of these organizations is presented in Table 12.3 and further information can be accessed through their Web sites.

ORGANIZATION/SOCIETY	WEB SITE
World Federation For Ultrasound in Medicine and Biology (WFUMB)	http://www.wfumb.org
European Federation of Societies for Ultrasound in Medicine and Biology (EFSUMB)	http://www.efsumb.org
British Medical Ultrasound Society (BMUS)	http://www.bmus.org
American Institute of Ultrasound in Medicine (AIUM)	http://www.aium.org
Australasian Society for Ultrasound in Medicine	http://www.asum.com.au

Table 12.3 List of ultrasound organizations and societies which offer safety guidelines

MACHINE CONTROLS WHICH INFLUENCE HAZARD

The exposure intensity and therefore any possible associated temperature rise are affected by many operator-dependent controls. The operator should understand the influence of the machine controls

Initial Power Setting/Output

Ultrasound machines are normally set up for all application-specific settings. This sets a default acoustic output which should be adequate to perform each examination. Application presets for obstetrics should default the machine's output to a low setting. The operator should only increase the output power setting if it is necessary and required to improve image quality.

Mode of Operation

B mode generally has the lowest power output and intensity. M mode, color flow imaging, and spectral Doppler have higher outputs which can cause more heating at the site of examination. Examinations should use B mode in the first instance and employ the use of color and spectral Doppler only when and if required.

Exposure Time

The overall examination should be kept as short as possible to obtain the required level of diagnostic information.

Stationary Probe

The probe should not be held in any fixed position for any longer than necessary. Operators should keep the transducer moving so that specific tissues are not subjected to long periods of stationary beam exposure. Use freeze frame and cineloop which allow images to be reviewed without continuing exposure.

Other Machine Controls

The intensity (and temperature rise) is highly dependent on other scanner settings such as:
- transmitted frequency used
- depth of examination
- focus.

The operator should be aware of and monitor changes to the values of TI and MI in response to changes in machine control settings and transducer combinations.

Table 12.4 summarizes the recommended guidelines issued by the British Medical Ultrasound Society (BMUS) in 2000 for thermal and mechanical indices. Full details of this can be accessed on their Web site.

EPIDEMIOLOGICAL EVIDENCE

Epidemiology is the study of how often diseases occur in different groups of people and why. A key feature of epidemiology is the measurement of disease outcomes in relation to a population at risk.

	BIOLOGICAL EFFECT	ACTION BY OPERATOR
MI > 0.3	Possibility of minor damage to neonatal lung or intestines	Reduce exposure times as much as possible
MI > 0.7	Theoretical risk of cavitation Risk of cavitation when conducting contrast agent studies	Reduce exposure times as much as possible
TI > 0.7	Increased risk of heating	Overall exposure time of an embryo or fetus should be restricted
TI > 1	Increased risk of heating	Eye scanning not recommended Overall exposure time of an embryo or fetus should be restricted
TI > 3	Significant risk of heating	Scanning of an embryo or fetus not recommended

Table 12.4 Recommended guidelines for values of MI and TI issued by BMUS

As a consequence of the rapid development of ultrasound as a diagnostic tool, the general population has been and is being exposed to more ultrasound energy than ever before. This is especially true for exposures of the fetus.

In the case of ultrasound, epidemiological studies have been used to search for risks associated with previous exposure to diagnostic ultrasound of fetuses (in utero) in early pregnancy as it is known that the developing human embryo or fetus is particularly sensitive to the ultrasound beam.

The outcomes of published epidemiology research evidence have suggested associations between ultrasound exposure and factors such as reduced birth weight, delayed speech development, dyslexia, and non-right handedness. However, some of this evidence has been conflicting and the reliability of these outcomes has since been questioned.

To date, diagnostic ultrasound has not been proved to be unsafe in humans. It is important to note that much of this research work was conducted before output levels were relaxed by the FDA in 1991 and that there is limited data for modern powerful diagnostic equipment using Doppler, harmonic imaging, and contrast agents. Ongoing research into bioeffects is necessary to reaffirm that ultrasound is still a safe modality.

Continuous vigilance is necessary, particularly in areas of concern such as the use of pulsed Doppler in the first trimester.

SUMMARY

- To date, diagnostic ultrasound has not been proved to be unsafe in humans
- Epidemiology data have several limitations:
  - Limited data for modern powerful diagnostic equipment
  - Ongoing research into bioeffects still necessary
  - Using pulsed Doppler, harmonic imaging, contrast agents
- Output regulations relaxed in 1991 for obstetric scans (> 7 times increase)
- Operator responsible for risk/benefit analysis
- Many machine controls have a significant effect
- Displayed MI and TI remove some guesswork for end users
- Knowledge, understanding, and training important
- Prudent use is practiced – ALARA principle
- Many guidelines offered to end users

References

Barnett SB (ed) 1998 Conclusions and recommendations on thermal and non thermal mechanisms for biological effects of ultrasound. WFUMB (World Federation for Ultrasound in Medicine and Biology) Symposium on Safety for Ultrasound in Medicine. Ultrasound in Medicine and Biology 24:1–55

Barnett SB, Kossoff G (eds) 1992 Issues and recommendations regarding thermal mechanisms for biological effects of ultrasound. WFUMB (World Federation for Ultrasound in Medicine and Biology) Symposium on Safety and Standardisation in Medical Ultrasound. Ultrasound in Medicine and Biology (special issue) 18

British Medical Ultrasound Society (BMUS) 2000 Guidelines for the safe use of diagnostic ultrasound equipment. Online. Available: www.bmus.org/ultras-safety/us-safety03.asp

Henderson J, Whittingham TA, Dunn T 1997 A review of the acoustical output of modern diagnostic ultrasound equipment. BMUS Bulletin 5:10–14

Quality assurance and performance testing

CONTENTS

LEARNING OBJECTIVES

1 Discuss the significance of ultrasound performance testing.

2 Explain what an ultrasound test phantom is.

3 List the acoustic properties of ultrasound test phantoms.

4 Explain why there are a number of test phantoms available.

5 Describe a number of performance tests that can be routinely carried out.

6 List some key limitations of performance testing.

INTRODUCTION

This chapter provides the reader with a general overview of quality assurance (QA) and performance testing of diagnostic ultrasound equipment. Performance testing of pulse-echo imaging systems will be covered, however because the evaluation of Doppler systems is technically more difficult and is normally performed by specialized medical physicists, it will not be included in this chapter.

QUALITY ASSURANCE

QA is the process of ensuring that all aspects of an ultrasound service meet and perform to agreed standards. The aim of QA is to maintain standards, and to seek to improve the performance of all aspects of an ultrasound service. QA is an essential aspect of clinical governance as it is a risk management tool for ensuring minimum standards of practice and performance are attained. This provides reassurance that all patients have access to high-quality ultrasound services wherever they are.

A comprehensive quality assurance programme should consider:
- the quality of the diagnostic investigation
- the quality of the patient service
- the quality of image production
- the maintenance of equipment.

The quality of the diagnostic investigation and patient service will be affected by factors such as operator training/competence and reporting procedures. These aspects will not be discussed here as this section will concentrate on the quality of image production specifically relating to the QA assessment and performance testing of diagnostic ultrasound machines.

While performance testing in X-ray modalities is almost universally practiced, in ultrasound, performance testing remains somewhat controversial for reasons which include:
- Ultrasound imaging is considered to be an established and safe modality
- Modern ultrasound scanners are considered very stable
- Ultrasound QA testing is often rather subjective
- There are no regulations requiring a QA program.

There are currently recommendations from the UK Department of Health and guidance from national and international bodies (such as the Institute of Physics and Engineering in Medicine and the American Institute of Ultrasound in Medicine) (see references) as to suggested measures and methods for QA testing. In the UK, only one clinical application, breast ultrasound imaging, has any formal mandatory requirements for the QA performance testing of ultrasound scanning equipment.

QUALITY ASSURANCE TESTING

Equipment Performance Testing

Ultrasound images are formed by transmitting and receiving ultrasound signals which are then processed by a number of individual components within an ultrasound machine. These components have different operations to perform before producing the images that we see on screen.

The accuracy with which the ultrasound image represents the anatomical area under investigation depends on the correct operation of these components and the accuracy of the various signal and image processing functions.

Many faults which can develop on ultrasound scanning equipment are not obvious to the user and gradual changes in performance are especially difficult to detect. Quantifiable assessment of a system's performance is therefore required to detect any deterioration at an early stage.

The goal of QA testing is to:
- ensure that an ultrasound system is set up correctly and performs to agreed standards
- maintain consistency of system performance
- provide early detection of problems.

The performance assessment and QA of diagnostic ultrasound scanners can also help to:
- inform the decision making process in the procurement and replacement of equipment
- assess new imaging modalities and signal processing techniques.

Ultrasound QA testing should provide objective, accurate, and repeatable measurement of the image displayed on the ultrasound screen, i.e. as seen by the operators. To be successful, QA testing should be easy to implement, simple to use, and able to detect faults at an early stage. It requires the use of strict protocols and documentation in order to ensure standardization of procedures.

In the UK, the Institute of Physics and Engineering in Medicine (IPEM) has produced guidelines for the routine QA of ultrasound imaging systems (Price 1995). The IPEM report advocates three levels of QA testing:
- Acceptance/baseline tests
- User tests
- Routine QA tests (carried out by third party).

Baseline acceptance tests

These tests should be carried out with any new machine and whenever a new probe or major hardware or software upgrade is added. Typically, it is carried out by a member of the medical physics department. It includes all the tests specified for routine QA, and establishes baseline readings for which further routine and user tests can be compared.

User tests

These are to be carried out at frequent intervals (between 1 to 4 weeks) by the operator, in order to discover any significant changes in scanner performance over time. It includes a number of simple tests which require a minimum amount of time to carry out. These tests relate to the aspects of the scanner function on which users depend for clinically meaningful results and include simple checks, such as testing caliper accuracy.

Routine QA tests

These are to be carried out by a third party, typically by a member of the medical physics department or possibly by a service engineer. They should be performed ideally every 6 months but at least every 12 months. These include a full range of tests which have relevance to normal clinical use and which are likely to detect deterioration in performance.

Equipment Required for Image Performance Testing

Tissue equivalent (TE) phantoms

There are a number of commercially available ultrasound devices that can be used to test whether an ultrasound system is operating correctly and consistently over time. These devices, known as test phantoms, are designed to have similar acoustic characteristics to those of soft tissue and should ideally be composed of material which allows:

- sound to travel at a speed of 1540 ms^{-1}
- attenuation of 0.5–0.8 dB/cm/MHz
- scattering properties similar to the echogenicity of soft tissue.

The tissue-like attenuation and echogenicity of tissue equivalent phantoms allows the testing of ultrasound systems using actual clinical settings.

Commercially available test phantoms are normally filled with an aqueous gel or are formed from urethane materials. They contain various targets and structures designed for testing a number of parameters. Examples of some commercially available test phantoms are illustrated in Figure 13.1.

Gel-based tissue equivalent phantoms consist of a closed container filled with an aqueous gel material loaded with graphite particles. These are designed to scatter ultrasound and produce an image that is similar to soft tissue, typically that of the liver. These phantoms have all the required acoustic characteristics matched for soft tissue as indicated above. The main disadvantage with this type of gel-filled phantom is that there is a tendency for the gel to dry out over time which potentially could change the tissue equivalent acoustic properties.

Polyurethane rubber-based phantoms, in comparison, are very stable and do not need to be totally enclosed to avoid them drying out. They can be made to have similar attenuation and scattering properties of soft tissue but have one distinct disadvantage in that the speed of sound is slower, 1450 ms^{-1} compared to 1540 ms^{-1} which an ultrasound machine is calibrated to. This discrepancy amounts to a 6–7% propagation speed error and becomes significant when testing caliper accuracy. The manufacturers have attempted to compensate for this by altering the position and distance of the internal targets within the phantom (positioning them closer together) so that these urethane phantoms can be used to test caliper measurements accurately.

Test phantoms contain a variety of structures and targets which can be used to test a range of imaging parameters. Figure 13.2 shows a typical arrangement of targets and structures for a general purpose test phantom. They contain groups of small nylon wires which can be used to measure image resolution and test distance accuracy. They also contain structures of varying sizes to mimic simple cysts. Some have structures which represent more complicated cysts designed to have a range of scattering patterns compared to the background tissue equivalent medium in order to assess contrast resolution and estimate the dynamic range.

Ultrasound images are formed using a variety of different transducers which operate over a range of frequencies and depths. Therefore ultrasound phantoms come in various shapes and sizes to accommodate this. If a low-frequency transducer is to be tested (2–5 MHz) then the test phantom will need to be relatively large and typically will need to be around 15 cm deep. For higher frequency transducers (7 MHz–12 MHz), where the beam is less penetrating but the images have improved resolution, then a smaller phantom is required with smaller structures to be able to assess and measure this. Two test phantoms which are designed for high- and low-frequency transducer applications can be seen in Figure 13.3.

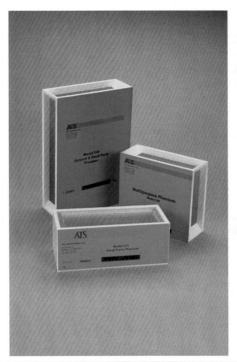

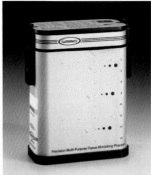

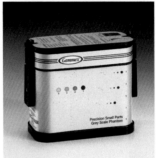

Fig. 13.1 • Examples of some commercially available test phantoms used for ultrasound QA performance testing (Reproduced with permission of Gammex.)

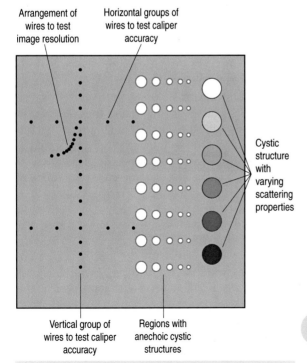

Arrangement of wires to test image resolution

Horizontal groups of wires to test caliper accuracy

Cystic structure with varying scattering properties

Vertical group of wires to test caliper accuracy

Regions with anechoic cystic structures

Fig. 13.2 • Typical arrangement of nylon wire targets, simple and complex cysts with a range of scattering properties within a general purpose test phantom

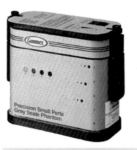

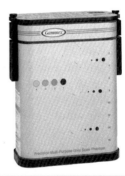

Fig. 13.3 • Two multi-purpose test phantoms. The larger phantom on the right-hand side is designed for transducers operating at low frequencies, typically between 2–5 MHz. The phantom on the left contains smaller structures and targets with smaller separation distances to test transducers operating at higher frequencies, typically above 5 MHz (Reproduced with permission of Gammex.)

WHAT PARAMETERS CAN BE MEASURED?

There are a number of imaging parameters that can be measured to assess and test the performance of a diagnostic ultrasound system. The most common, which will be discussed in this chapter, include:

1 testing measurement accuracy
2 testing image resolution
3 testing depth of penetration (sensitivity)
4 assessing dynamic range.

1. Testing Measurement Accuracy

Taking measurements is an essential part of inter-preting ultrasound scans and is fundamental to monitoring and assessing fetal growth, for exam-ple, and in differentiating normal anatomy from pathology. Ultrasound machines use electronic calipers to make measurements of structures to calculate linear distances, circumferences, and areas from frozen B-mode images.

Testing the measurement accuracy of a diagnos-tic ultrasound system can be easily undertaken by the end user by using an appropriate test phan-tom. It is usual to assess measurement accuracy in the vertical and horizontal planes even though clinically linear measurements can be taken at any angle within the ultrasound image.

Vertical measurements, which are made along the axis of the ultrasound beam, are assessed by acquiring an image of a vertical set of evenly spaced wires at a known separation within the ultrasound test phantom. Two of the wires are selected and the distance is measured using the electronic cali-pers, as illustrated in Figure 13.4. This electronic caliper measurement can then be compared to the known actual distance between the wires and can be expressed as a percentage error.

Horizontal measurements can be assessed by selecting two targets on a horizontal row of evenly spaced wires within the test phantom, as illu-strated in Figure 13.5. Again, the measured dis-tance can be compared with the known actual distance and expressed as a percentage error using the simple equation below:

Percentage error =
$$\frac{\text{Actual measurement} - \text{Electronic measurement}}{\text{Actual measurement}} \times 100$$

Vertical and horizontal caliper measurements are affected by different factors. Vertical accuracy is determined by factors such as the speed of sound within the phantom whereas horizontal measure-ments are affected by other geometrical factors. Generally vertical (axial) measurements are more accurate than lateral measurements. Errors in

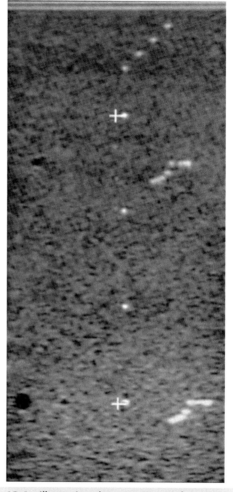

Fig. 13.4 · Illustrating the assessment of vertical measurements using a typical tissue equivalent phantom

either measurement of more than 2% are consid-ered as unacceptable.

Greater accuracy is achieved by measuring dis-tances between two wires which are positioned furthest apart rather than two which are only a couple of centimeters apart.

Circumference and area measurements are more difficult to assess and are usually conducted during routine QA testing which is normally performed by a medical physicist rather than the end user. Errors of more than 5% should be investigated.

2. Testing Image Resolution

Image resolution, referred to as spatial resolution, is defined as the ability of an ultrasound system to

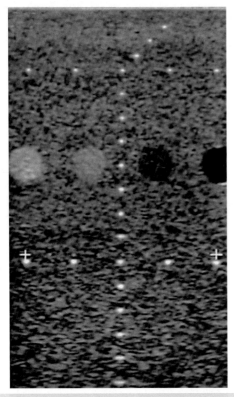

Fig. 13.5 • Illustrating the assessment of horizontal measurements using an appropriate test phantom

separate images which lie perpendicular or side by side to the ultrasound beam at the same depth from the transducer. Lateral resolution depends on the beam width, focusing characteristics of the transducer, number of displayed scan lines, and the system's sensitivity and gain settings. The best lateral resolution is achieved at the focal point where the ultrasound beam is narrowest.

There are two ways of testing axial and lateral resolution:
a) Object separation method
b) Single wire method.

These tests are normally performed by a medical physicist rather than the end user.

a) Object separation method

Most test phantoms contain a set of targets at different depths designed for the assessment of axial and lateral resolution which consist of a set of wires separated by decreasing vertical and horizontal spacing. An example is illustrated in Figure 13.6. The spacing of vertical wires to assess axial resolution decreases from a maximum separation distance of 2 mm to a minimum separation of 0.25 mm. In contrast, the spacing of horizontal target wires to assess lateral resolution is larger, ranging from a maximum separation of 5 mm to a minimum separation distance of 1.5 mm. This takes into account that lateral resolution is generally poorer than axial resolution in most imaging systems.

The system's axial and lateral resolution are determined by identifying the set of two resolvable wires with the smallest separation. Figure 13.7 shows an image of a test phantom with such an arrangement of wires. It can be seen that the ultrasound system is able to resolve all targets along the vertical axis (axial plane) but is unable to resolve targets separated by a distance less than 2.5 mm across the image (lateral plane).

The main disadvantage with this technique is that the measurement values are limited to the

distinguish two closely spaced targets as separate objects (see Chapter 7 on Resolution). If a system has poor resolution capabilities, small structures lying close to each other will appear as one object, causing incorrect interpretation of the ultrasound image. Spatial resolution can be divided into two main components in the scan plane, namely axial and lateral resolution.

Testing axial and lateral resolution

Axial resolution is the ability of an ultrasound system to distinguish two closely spaced targets as separate images along the axis of the ultrasound beam. Axial resolution depends on the transducer's operating frequency, damping characteristics, and spatial pulse length. Generally, the higher the frequency, the better the system's axial resolution. Axial resolution is generally superior to lateral resolution.

Lateral resolution is the ability of an ultrasound system to distinguish two closely spaced targets as

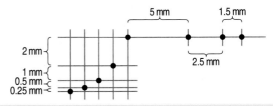

Fig. 13.6 • Showing a typical arrangement of wire spacing to assess axial and lateral resolution

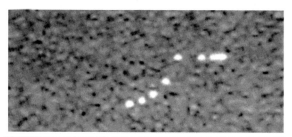

Fig. 13.7 • An image of a test phantom assessing axial and lateral resolution at a specific depth

spacing of targets within the test phantom and it is sometimes difficult to decide whether or not a pair of targets is resolved.

b) Single wire method

Using this method, any set of target wires can be chosen. Typically, the vertical set of target wires used to assess vertical distance are ideally suited for this (see Fig. 13.4).

The axial and lateral resolution is measured indirectly by measuring the length and width of individual wire targets at different depths corresponding to the transducer's near, mid, and far field range. Figures 13.8 and 13.9 illustrate this method for measuring image resolution using a single wire target.

Using this single wire method, the image of the target is magnified using the machine's zoom control facility to ensure that the errors when taking these small measurements are minimized. The main disadvantage of this technique is that it is

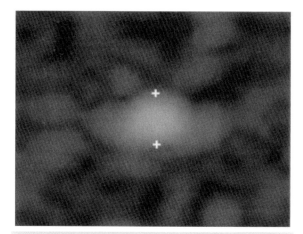

Fig. 13.8 • Assessment of axial resolution using a single wire method

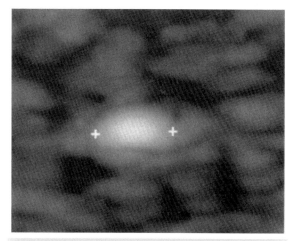

Fig. 13.9 • Assessment of lateral resolution using the single wire method

sometimes difficult to identify and determine the edges of these blurred target wires.

3. Testing Depth of Penetration (Sensitivity)

Also known as sensitivity, this is the ability of the ultrasound system to detect and display low-amplitude echoes and refers to the depth at which the deepest echo signal within an image can be detected and clearly displayed by the ultrasound system.

Clinically, echoes received from small structures deep within the tissue are very weak due to the attenuation of the propagating ultrasound beam. The ability of an ultrasound system to detect, display, and differentiate these weak echoes from background noise is extremely important in the interpretation of the ultrasound image.

The point in the image where this is reached is known as the maximum penetration depth. The penetration depth is affected by a number of factors which include:
- output power
- receiver gain
- transducer frequency and efficiency
- focusing
- signal processing within the ultrasound machine.

Measurement of penetration depth is useful and should be consistent over time. A loss in penetration depth, which can lead to a decrease in performance, can indicate a fault in one of the above factors.

For meaningful and comparative assessments, this test is performed using exactly the same settings for a given transducer. These are normally performed using a test phantom with the machine operating at maximum output power and using a deep focal zone setting to obtain a measurement of the maximum penetration depth. Figure 13.10 shows a typical image using the recommended set-up to test the penetration depth. The maximum depth at which scattering echoes can be detected and differentiated from background electronic noise is determined and measured using the electronic calipers.

4. Assessing Dynamic Range

Dynamic range refers to the way that the gray scale information is compressed into a usable range for display on the monitor and is the ratio of the largest signal to the smallest. This ratio is usually expressed on a decibel scale (dB). Clinically, gray scale processing and displayed dynamic range allow echoes of varying degrees of amplitude to be displayed in the same image. A broader or wider dynamic range yields more shades of gray, while a smaller or narrower dynamic range results in a more black and white or more contrasted appearance of the image.

The gray scale processing and therefore dynamic range of an ultrasound system can be assessed by using a suitable test phantom which typically consists of a group of targets which have varying contrasts relative to the background. An example of a typical test phantom is shown in Figure 13.11, and consists of a number of cylinders (which are imaged in cross-section) filled with a material of different scattering strengths to create areas of known and varying gray levels and echogenicity. Figure 13.12 shows an image using such a phantom to assess a system's dynamic range. This is estimated from the difference between the brightest and darkest regions which can be imaged simultaneously.

ELECTRICAL AND MECHANICAL SAFETY

Equipment-related physical checks should also be included in any ultrasound QA testing program and include regular visual inspection of:

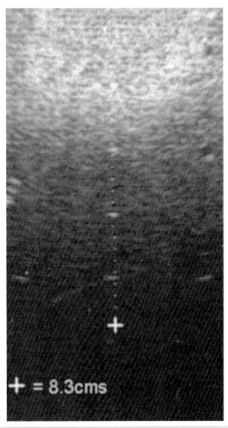

Fig. 13.10 • Measurement of penetration depth. Electronic caliper indicates the maximum penetration depth determined by the operator

+ = 8.3cms

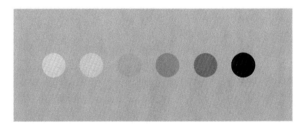

Fig. 13.11 • A typical phantom to test dynamic range which consists of a range of cylinders filled with materials of different scattering strengths compared to the background material

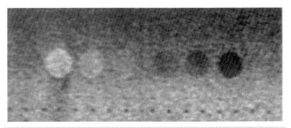

Fig. 13.12 • Ultrasound image using such a test phantom to assess dynamic range

- transducers, for cracks and delamination in the plastic housing
- cables, for any loose and frayed electrical cables
- peripherals
- air filters, ensuring that they are clean and not obstructed.

LIMITATIONS OF ULTRASOUND QA TESTING

A substantial effort has been made to determine the most appropriate and clinically relevant tests, with recommendations by many professional bodies who have published general guidelines describing standard methods for measuring the performance of ultrasound systems. These outline the most appropriate imaging tests, i.e. parameters that should be tested, the frequency of this testing, and the most appropriate phantoms to use. However, there are many machine controls and variables that must be considered which, on modern ultrasound systems, are difficult to individually control without affecting each other. This makes a clinically meaningful assessment regarding the performance of the ultrasound system using test phantoms subjective and difficult to quantify. To obtain optimum and reproducible results, it is important to take a rational and consistent approach to the ultrasound system's settings.

A straightforward approach adopted by the end user should include some basic tests such as checking caliper accuracy and measuring the depth of penetration, for example. These are extremely useful to monitor the performance of an ultrasound system.

Recent developments in technology leading to the use of higher frequency transducers with improved image resolution, for example, have improved the performance of ultrasound equipment to such an extent that many machines are now able to resolve targets on current phantoms easily. There is therefore a growing need for a new generation of test phantoms in order to measure adequately the capabilities of new equipment.

Further developments in ultrasound performance testing and phantoms are necessary and should lead to a standard practice of QA in all ultrasound departments in the future. As end users, we need to ensure that the equipment we use is adequate and appropriate to ensure high-quality diagnostic ultrasound imaging is achieved and maintained.

SUMMARY

- Test phantoms are made to contain various tissue equivalent materials
- Phantoms come in a variety of shapes and sizes
- Phantoms are utilized for a range of QA performance testing
- The guidelines for ultrasound QA performance testing programs are currently descriptive rather than prescriptive
- Maintaining an ultrasound QA testing program is straightforward and is effective in identifying deficiencies
- Guidelines need to be updated periodically as ultrasound technology develops

---

References

American Institute of Ultrasound in Medicine 1995 Quality assurance manual for gray scale ultrasound scanners (Stage 2). AIUM, Laurel, Maryland

Price R (ed) 1995 Institute of Physics and Engineering in Medicine Report 71: Routine quality assurance of ultrasound imaging systems. IPEM, York

Further reading

American College of Radiology 1999 ACR Technical standard for diagnostic medical physics performance monitoring of real time B-mode ultrasound equipment. ACR, Reston, Virginia

Goodsitt MM, Carson PL, Witt S et al (eds) 1998 Report of AAPM Ultrasound Task Group No 1: Real-time B-mode ultrasound quality control test procedures. Medical Physics 25 (8):1385–1406

Madsen E (ed) 1995 Quality assurance manual for gray scale ultrasound scanners (Stage 2). AIUM, Laurel, Maryland

Medical Devices Agency 1999 Evaluation Report MDA/98/52. HMSO, London

New technology and recent advances in ultrasound imaging

14

CONTENTS

LEARNING OBJECTIVES

1 Explain the principles behind the advances in technology described.

2 Describe the advantages of the advances in technology.

3 Describe any disadvantages in introducing the new technology.

4 Give examples of clinical applications of new technology.

In this chapter we shall look at some of the innovations in ultrasound imaging that have been introduced in the last five to ten years, and also some of the new technology which is still at the research and development stage.

DIGITAL BEAM FORMING

The beam former is the system of electronics that determines the shape of the beam. Earlier beam formers used either analog electronics or a combination of analog and digital electronics. In modern transducers the beam former is totally digital which enables the ultrasound beam to be focused with greater precision.

The amount of focusing and the position of the focus in an ultrasound beam is a function of the beam former. Focusing is achieved by applying delays to the inner elements of the group of crystals that are used to produce a composite ultrasound pulse and to receive echoes from the subject. Accurate timing of these delays is critical in producing a narrow beam focusing at the correct depth. In addition, the more accurate the timing of the delays, the less noise is produced and the better the contrast resolution.

Using analog beam formers, it is not possible to produce delay timers with the accuracy required and this limits their performance. However, beam formers are now produced using digital electronics for the time delays. In addition to producing narrower beams, digital beam formers can operate at higher frequencies and can be used with broad-bandwidth transducers.

HIGH-FREQUENCY IMAGING

High-frequency ultrasound imaging using frequencies above 20 MHz is being developed to enable the imaging of superficial structures at a very high resolution. Using conventional medical ultrasound at 5 MHz, it is possible to penetrate up to 20 cm and achieve a spatial resolution of 0.5–1.0 mm. However, with high-frequency ultrasound it is possible to image with a resolution of 50 microns ($\frac{1}{20}$ mm). The disadvantage is that because the attenuation is increased at high frequencies, penetration is reduced to a few millimeters.

The initial clinical applications of high-frequency ultrasound include the anterior chamber of the eye, intravascular ultrasound of arterial walls, skin, and cartilage.

EXTENDED FIELD OF VIEW IMAGING

This is an imaging process which combines static B-mode techniques with real-time imaging so that a large subject area can be viewed on a single static image. Extended field of view (FOV) images are obtained by sliding the probe over the area of interest and as the images are acquired they are 'stitched together' electronically (Fig. 14.1). The result is a single slice image covering the whole area of interest, for example a full length view of the Achilles tendon (Fig. 14.2). Image feature recognition software is used to combine images.

This feature is now standard on most current ultrasound systems, and is particularly beneficial where large areas of the patient need to be visualized on one image, such as obstetrics or musculoskeletal imaging.

COMPOUND IMAGING

This technique combines electronic beam steering with conventional linear array technology to produce real-time images acquired from different view angles (see Fig. 14.3) Between 3 and 9 sector images are rapidly acquired and combined to produce a compound real-time image (see Fig. 14.4). Compound imaging improves image quality by reducing speckle, clutter, and other acoustic artifacts. It also gives better definition of the boundaries of structures. Because of the improved contrast resolution, compound imaging may be useful for the breast, peripheral blood vessels, and musculoskeletal applications.

THREE-DIMENSIONAL IMAGING

In conventional two-dimensional imaging the operator integrates a large number of images representing slices of the subject to form a mental

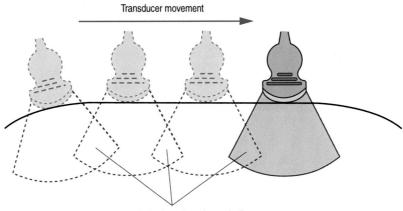
Transducer movement

Images stitched together electronically

Fig. 14.1 • Diagram showing how images of the subject are acquired before being electronically 'stitched together'

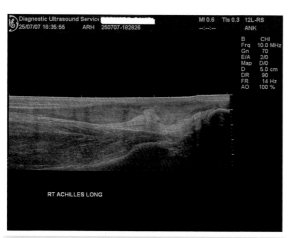

Fig. 14.2 • Extended field image showing the full length of the Achilles tendon

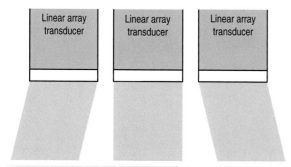

Fig. 14.3 • Diagram showing how electronic beam steering is used to acquire images from different angles

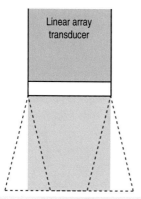

Fig. 14.4 • Diagram showing how the images are combined to produce a compound real-time image

3-D image of the subject's anatomy; however this mental 3-D picture is only available to the operator and only during the scanning process. The challenge for equipment designers is to produce a 3-D image which can be reviewed after the examination by the operator and also by other staff and patients. With 3-D ultrasound, an image of the surface of a structure is produced; this can be rotated through different planes and the surface viewed from many angles. It is also possible for the operator to 'peel away' layers of a 3-D image and see inside the structure.

3-D Imaging Technology

The production of a 3-D image requires a volume of tissue to be scanned. The data from this volume are then used to construct the types of image required. There are three approaches to scanning a volume of tissue: free-hand, mechanical, and electronic scanning.

Free-hand 3-D imaging

In this approach the operator sweeps the probe across the volume of interest and a series of scanning planes are recorded according to their position on the patient (see Fig. 14.5). In order to register these planes, a method of determining the position of the transducer in space is required.

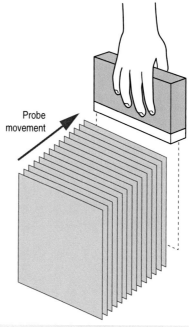

Fig. 14.5 • In free-hand 3-D imaging the operator sweeps the probe across the volume of interest

113

This can be achieved by using a receiver in the probe which will detect a magnetic field generated by a transmitter situated next to the couch (see Fig 14.6). Each image slice will have image information and position information for use in 3-D construction. Another method of determining the position of the scan plane is to use a radio transmitter and radio detection coils attached to the probe.

The advantage of free-hand 3-D imaging is that a large volume can be scanned, however considerable skill is required and any measurements made are not as accurate as the automated scanning methods.

Mechanical 3-D imaging

In a mechanical system the probe is attached to a motor which mechanically oscillates in a sector movement at right angles to the imaging plane (see Fig. 14.7). A volume of tissue is scanned with 2-D image data collected at regularly spaced intervals and stored for 3-D construction. In addition to the sector volume already described, parallel slice volumes (see Fig. 14.8) and rotational slice volumes are also available. The parallel slice method gives the most accurate reconstruction because the slices are equally spaced; however the scanning mechanisms are more bulky than the sector and rotational methods. With the sector and rotational volume methods, the separation between the slices increases with distance from the axis of rotation causing a decrease in resolution and less accurate 3-D reconstruction.

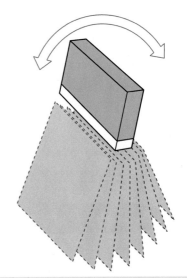

Fig. 14.7 • Diagram showing how the probe oscillates in a sector movement to scan a volume of tissue

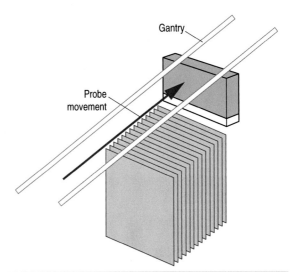

Fig. 14.8 • Diagram showing how a parallel slice volume is scanned in mechanical 3-D imaging

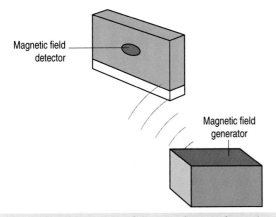

Fig. 14.6 • The position of the transducer is determined by scanning within a magnetic field. A receiver in the transducer detects the magnetic field

Electronic 3-D imaging and 4-D imaging

This approach makes use of a transducer with a 2-D array (see Fig. 14.9) with the data being collected from a pyramid shaped volume. This type of transducer may have over 2000 elements and collects the data from each image plane simultaneously. This enables the transducer to scan over 20 volumes per second and produce real-time 3-D images – this is known as 4-D imaging.

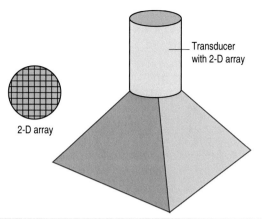

Fig. 14.9 • Diagram showing a transducer with a 2-D array of piezoelectric elements, which collects data from a pyramid shaped volume

HARMONIC IMAGING

The aim of this method of ultrasound imaging is to reduce haze or scatter, and produce a cleaner image with higher contrast resolution. This technology takes advantage of a process known as non-linear propagation where ultrasound transmitted at the fundamental frequency is transferred into the harmonic frequencies. For example, if the fundamental frequency is 3 MHz, some of the energy would be transferred to the second harmonic (6 MHz) and third harmonic (9 MHz) frequencies, and to higher harmonics.

In harmonic imaging a broad bandwidth transducer (see Fig. 14.10) is used to transmit ultrasound at the fundamental frequency (see Fig. 14.11) and detect echoes at both the second harmonic and fundamental frequencies (see Figs 14.12 and 14.13).

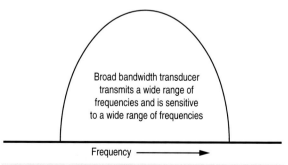

Fig. 14.10 • Frequency spectrum of a broad bandwidth transducer, which shows the range of frequencies the transducer is able to transmit and the range of frequencies it is sensitive to

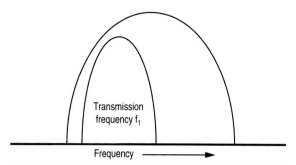

Fig. 14.11 • Diagram showing the transmitted frequency spectrum (fundamental frequency) compared with the total range of frequencies available to the broad bandwidth transducer

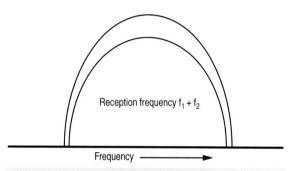

Fig. 14.12 • Diagram showing the frequency spectrum detected by the transducer

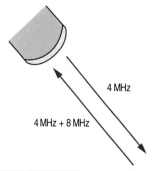

Fig. 14.13 • The transducer transmits fundamental frequency ultrasound and receives both fundamental frequency and 2nd harmonic frequency ultrasound

However, the signals produced by the fundamental frequency are filtered out and not used to form the image (see Fig. 14.14). The advantage of this method of imaging is that the second harmonic frequency contains the high amplitude echoes which arise from the axis of the beam whereas the fundamental frequency contains the low amplitude artifactual echoes and these are filtered out.

115

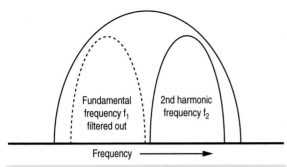

Fig. 14.14 • Diagram showing the fundamental frequency spectrum filtered out leaving the 2nd harmonic frequency spectrum for producing the image

Higher acoustic power is required and, because of the narrower range of frequencies used for image formation, pulse lengths are longer than in fundamental imaging. This results in poorer axial resolution.

This method of imaging is advantageous when scanning through large depths of tissue and is also used in conjunction with micro-bubble contrast agents. The facility is now available on most systems, however it may prove beneficial to de-activate the function during certain examinations when no perceivable benefit is obtained.

CONTRAST AGENTS

Contrast agents are used in medical imaging to increase contrast and make organs, vessels, and body cavities easier to see. In medical ultrasound contrast agents containing micro-bubbles have been found to give the highest contrast.

The micro-bubbles consist of air or inert gas encapsulated in a layer of protein or polymer. This layer prevents the bubbles dissolving too rapidly in blood or coalescing to form larger bubbles. The micro-bubbles are typically 3 μm in diameter, a similar size to red blood cells, and can therefore be transported into the smallest capillaries and across the lungs. It is important that they can survive the passage across the lungs because this enables imaging of the arterial system using a venous injection.

The micro-bubbles produce strong scattering because of the large acoustic impedance difference at the gas/blood interface. This scattering is further enhanced by the bubbles in a sound wave resonating (oscillating) at a specific frequency according to their diameter and therefore acting as a producer as well as a reflector of sound. This frequency is in the MHz range, approximately the same as the transducer frequency, and is therefore detected by the transducer.

Ultrasound contrast agents are used in a variety of clinical situations such as cardiovascular imaging to image blood vessels; gynecological imaging to image the uterine cavity and patency of the fallopian tubes; and to quantify the flow characteristics through an organ or tumor by producing wash-in/wash-out curves. Many of these examinations are now in routine use within many departments, and greatly assisting in the diagnosis of a range of conditions.

Targeted Micro-bubbles

Targeted micro-bubbles are being developed, which have special characteristics which bind them to certain cells such as inflamed cells or cancer cells. The aim is to develop a non-invasive method of imaging diseased organs. Work is also being carried out to research the possibility of using these targeted micro-bubbles to deliver drugs or genetic material, by disrupting them when they reach areas of pathology.

Contrast Agents and Harmonic Imaging

When micro-bubbles are insonated they resonate at their fundamental frequency and also at their second, third, and higher harmonic frequencies. By using harmonic imaging tuned to the second harmonic frequency of the micro-bubbles, it is possible to discriminate between the micro-bubbles and tissue. This technique increases the contrast between the micro-bubbles and normal tissue.

The contrast can be further enhanced by using pulse inversion imaging – see below.

PULSE INVERSION IMAGING

This imaging modality is used to increase the sensitivity of ultrasound to contrast agents. In conventional B-mode or harmonic imaging, only one pulse of ultrasound at a time is transmitted. In pulse inversion imaging, two pulses are transmitted, the second being an inverted copy of the first

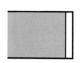 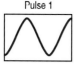 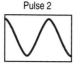

Pulses 180º out of phase

Fig. 14.15 • Diagram showing two pulses being transmitted from the transducer, the second pulse being an inverted copy of the first pulse

one (see Fig. 14.15). When the echoes from these two pulses are detected by the transducer they are added together.

Echoes reflected from normal tissues cancel each other out when they are added after detection (see Fig. 14.16). However, echoes from micro-bubbles do not cancel each other out because of the harmonic frequencies produced by the bubbles (see Figs 14.17 and 14.18). This results in an ultrasound image where the contrast produced by the micro-bubbles is significantly enhanced. It is particularly useful in small vessels where the

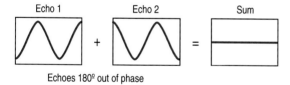

Echoes 180º out of phase

Fig. 14.16 • Diagram showing how echoes reflected from normal tissues cancel each other out when they are added

bubbles are moving slowly, and therefore do not move far between successive transmitted pulses.

An advantage of pulse inversion imaging over harmonic imaging is that it is possible to use a wide range of frequencies for transmission and detection of ultrasound. This results in a shorter pulse length and therefore improved axial resolution.

ELASTOGRAPHY

Elastography is the measurement of the elastic properties of tissue, and ultrasound can be used for this purpose. It uses echo information to produce a 2-D display of the elasticity (stiffness) of tissues scanned. The elasticity of tissue is determined by applying stress, and measuring any associated movement. The stiffness of the tissues is not necessarily related to its backscatter properties, and may therefore result in contrast between tissues which is not apparent with conventional ultrasound imaging. Software in the ultrasound machine measures the degree of compression of tissue and calculates the elasticity.

The main application of elastography is in differentiating between benign and malignant tissue, malignant tissues being less elastic and therefore harder to compress than benign tissue. This technique has been used to look at breast tumors, where the tumor is imaged by ultrasound before and after compression by the probe. Elastography has also been used to examine prostate tumors

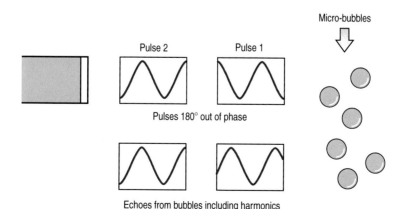

Fig. 14.17 • Diagram showing echoes reflected from micro-bubbles (these echoes include some harmonic frequencies)

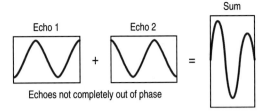

Fig. 14.18 • Diagram showing how the echoes from micro-bubbles, because they are not completely out of phase, result in a high-amplitude signal when added

and the elasticity of arterial walls; however the technique is still in its infancy and is largely used as a research tool.

TISSUE CHARACTERIZATION

Tissue characterization using ultrasound has been the goal of scientists for many years. If successful it would produce quantifiable information about the type of tissue being imaged, similar to the Hounsfield units obtained during computerized tomography (CT) scanning. The aim is to analyze the signals received from different tissues and characterize them according to their acoustic properties. However, the transmitted pulse and the echoes from the site of interest are affected by the intervening tissue, which gives a distorted signal and, until this problem is dealt with satisfactorily, tissue characterization will remain the subject of research.

TISSUE MOTION

Conventional B-mode ultrasound scanning will provide information on overall tissue motion. To obtain more information on internal tissue motions of organs, a method known as Doppler tissue imaging (DTI) has been developed. This is a variation of color Doppler imaging and can be implemented using a decreased wall thump filter to record low velocities and decrease signals from the movement of blood, in order to retain only the stronger tissue signal in the image. The technique is still in the research phase, but has the potential to provide useful information in the diagnosis of pathology of organs, particularly the heart.

PORTABLE ULTRASOUND MACHINES

Portable machines have been available since the mid 1990s. These machines were similar in size to a portable television set and were fairly limited in the range of applications offered and their performance. However, the advances in flat screen and microprocessor technology has meant that there are now laptop machines which have a range of applications and image quality approaching that of conventional scanners. In addition to this there are inexpensive handheld scanners which have applications in emergency investigations such as FAST (focused abdominal sonography for trauma) scanning.

SUMMARY

- Digital beam forming improves lateral resolution by accurately focusing the ultrasound beam

- High-frequency imaging uses frequencies above the normal diagnostic range (above 20 MHz) to produce very high resolution ultrasound images of superficial structures

- Extended field of view is an ultrasound technique which enables the operator to produce a static image of a large section

- Compound imaging improves contrast resolution by scanning from multiple view angles

- Three approaches to 3-D scanning are described: free hand, mechanical, and electronic scanning. With electronic scanning it is possible to produce real-time 3-D images

- Harmonic imaging reduces haze and scatter when scanning large patients. This is achieved by using only second harmonic frequency echoes to produce the image

- The main contrast agent used in ultrasound imaging is a solution containing micro-bubbles of air or inert gas. These micro-bubbles are of a similar size to red blood cells, which enables them to cross the lungs. This enables them to be used for arterial studies using a venous injection

- The visualization of contrast agents can be improved by using harmonic imaging or pulse inversion imaging

- Elastography is a technique under development, which attempts to distinguish malignant tissue from normal tissue by measuring the amount that a structure distorts under pressure. Ultrasound imaging is used to make the measurement

- The aim of tissue characterization is to analyze the signals received from different tissues and characterize them according to their acoustic properties. This technology is still in the research stage with many difficulties to overcome

- Tissue motion imaging is a development of color Doppler and is used to look at the movement of tissues within body organs such as the heart

- Portable ultrasound machines have undergone major improvements over the last 10 years and the better machines perform almost as well as conventional scanners

MULTIPLE CHOICE QUESTIONS

Select all the correct answers in the following:

The Ultrasound Beam

1 An ultrasound beam passing through the body
   a. is attenuated
   b. produces heating of tissues
   c. can be reflected
   d. produces ionization

2 Ultrasonic pulses
   a. are poorly transmitted by liquids
   b. are poorly transmitted by air gaps
   c. are partially reflected at interfaces between two liquid media
   d. are partially transmitted at interfaces between two solid media

3 The Fraunhofer zone is the
   a. image plane
   b. image focus
   c. near field
   d. far field

4 Which of the following statements are true concerning the nature of diagnostic ultrasound in liver?
   a. The wave speed and frequency are constant regardless of the wavelength
   b. The wave speed is constant regardless of the wavelength
   c. Wave speed increases with the increasing frequency
   d. None of the above

5 Which of the following characteristics of diagnostic ultrasound applies also to X-radiation?
   a. It is a wave phenomenon
   b. Its wave speed and frequency are inversely proportional

   c. Matter must be present for transmission
   d. Molecular compression and rarefaction occur

6 When two or more (plane) ultrasound waves exist in the same medium at the same time
   a. they will interfere constructively if traveling with the same direction and phase
   b. standing waves will be produced if they are traveling with the same direction and phase
   c. standing waves will be produced if they are traveling in the same direction but out of phase
   d. None of the above

7 Specific acoustic impedance as applied to diagnostic ultrasound increases with increasing
   a. frequency
   b. wavelength
   c. mass
   d. density

8 When the diagnostic ultrasound beam is incident on the surface separating different tissues
   a. none of the beam will be transmitted
   b. none of the beam will be reflected
   c. reflection can occur when the beam is at right angles to the interface
   d. when incident at greater than the critical angle, there will be total transmission

9 When an acoustic wave is transmitted through soft tissue
   a. there will be no reduction in intensity
   b. attenuation will occur
   c. energy will be transmitted by way of ionization and excitation
   d. energy will be transmitted by way of Compton scattering

10 When an ultrasound beam is attenuated while passing through tissue
  a. a 3 dB loss is equivalent to a 50% reduction in intensity
  b. a 6 dB loss is equivalent to a 100% reduction in intensity
  c. the normal rate is 10 dB/cm/MHz
  d. 90% reduction of the original intensity is equivalent to a 90 dB loss

11 When a transmitted ultrasound beam changes direction across an interface, this is called
  a. reflection
  b. defraction
  c. refraction
  d. scattering

12 Ultrasound and X-rays differ in which of the following ways?
  a. One is transverse, the other longitudinal
  b. One requires matter, the other does not
  c. One has constant wave speed, the other variable wave speed (in soft tissue)
  d. All of the above

13 Diagnostic ultrasound intensity is often measured in
  a. W/cm^2
  b. grays
  c. rad
  d. decibels

14 Intensity is equal to
  a. power/area
  b. area/power
  c. amplitude/distance
  d. frequency/wavelength

15 Diagnostic ultrasound intensity
  a. increases with increasing frequency
  b. is a measure of particle displacement in the conduction medium
  c. is measured in mW/cm^2
  d. is the same as ultrasound power

16 As ultrasound is transmitted through tissue, its intensity decreases because of
  a. excitation
  b. absorption
  c. scattering
  d. divergence

17 Acoustic reflectivity
  a. is determined by acoustic impedance at an interface
  b. equals 100 if $Z_1 = Z_2$
  c. is higher for an air–soft-tissue interface than a bone–soft-tissue interface
  d. increases with increasing frequency

18 An ultrasound wave may be described as
  a. a longitudinal pressure wave
  b. a transverse wave
  c. being formed by particle oscillations
  d. changes in electrical properties of tissues

19 Ultrasound used for diagnosis
  a. has a frequency in the region 2 to 10 kHz
  b. has a velocity in air of 1500 ms^{-1}
  c. will not travel through a vacuum
  d. is produced and detected by a transducer

20 Ultrasound has the following properties. It
  a. can be deflected by a magnetic field
  b. is attenuated in tissue
  c. has a sinusoidal wave form
  d. can travel through water

21 An ultrasound beam is attenuated
  a. by reflection at a tissue interface
  b. and causes ionization of atoms
  c. by scattering
  d. by absorption in tissues

22 Greater than 50% energy reflection will take place at a
  a. soft-tissue–bone interface
  b. water–soft-tissue interface
  c. soft-tissue–gas interface
  d. muscle–fat interface

23 The magnitude of the reflected signal
  a. decreases as the angle of incidence approaches 90 degrees
  b. depends on the change of acoustic impedance at an interface
  c. is independent of the acoustic impedance
  d. depends on the frequency of the beam

24 Interference phenomena
  a. may occur when two waves interact
  b. are more common with continuous wave ultrasound

c. always produce a wave form of reduced amplitude

d. may be of value to ultrasound

25 Acoustic impedance depends on
   a. the intensity of the ultrasound beam
   b. the elasticity of the tissue
   c. tissue density
   d. tissue temperature

26 In which of the following materials is the speed of ultrasound greatest?
   a. Air
   b. Bone
   c. Water
   d. Soft tissue

27 What is the wavelength of a 5 MHz ultrasound pulse in soft tissue?
   a. 0.3 mm
   b. 0.5 mm
   c. 3 mm
   d. 5 mm

28 As frequency increases
   a. wavelength increases
   b. imaging depth decreases
   c. propagation speed decreases
   d. a and b

29 The frequency of a sound wave is determined by
   a. the media through which it travels
   b. its propagation
   c. its source
   d. reflection

30 As frequency increases, the attenuation coefficient
   a. decreases
   b. increases
   c. stays the same
   d. attenuation coefficient not affected by frequency

31 Which of the following sound frequencies would include diagnostic ultrasound?
   a. 10 Hz
   b. 10 kHz
   c. 100 kHz
   d. 10 MHz

32 Velocity of ultrasound
   a. depends on the transmitted frequency
   b. varies for different materials

c. is temperature dependent
d. is equal for muscle and bone

33 The velocity of an ultrasound beam may be determined by measuring the
   a. time taken for a pulse to be returned through a Perspex block of a known thickness
   b. time taken for a pulse to be returned through a known depth of water
   c. reflection of the beam by a wire mesh placed in water
   d. distance between peaks of the wave form

34 The propagation speed of sound through soft tissue is
   a. 1450 ms^{-1}
   b. 1650 ms^{-1}
   c. 1540 ms^{-1}
   d. 1230 cms^{-1}

35 Given the various physical characteristics of ultrasound, then it is true that
   a. its speed is the same in all materials
   b. its speed does not depend on its frequency
   c. its speed depends on the density of the supporting medium
   d. its speed increases with frequency

36 Lateral resolution can be improved by
   a. damping
   b. pulsing
   c. focusing
   d. reflecting

37 Axial resolution can be improved by
   a. damping
   b. pulsing
   c. focusing
   d. increasing operating frequency

38 The resolution of an ultrasound beam may be determined by
   a. imaging a series of wires at varying depth from the transducer face
   b. imaging a series of wires all the same depth from the transducer face
   c. compound scanning around a Perspex block containing a single central wire
   d. linear scanning of a single wire in a water bath

39 The lateral resolution of the diagnostic ultrasound system is
a. also called the azimuthal resolution
b. determined by the slice thickness
c. better with higher frequency
d. better than axial resolution

40 The axial resolution of a transducer is primarily determined by
a. spatial pulse length
b. the transducer diameter
c. the acoustic impedance of tissue
d. density

41 The lateral resolution of a transducer is primarily determined by
a. spatial pulse length
b. the beam width
c. the acoustic impedance of tissue
d. applied voltage

The Transducer

1 The fundamental operating principle of medical ultrasound transducers is
a. Snell's law
b. ALARA principle
c. piezoelectric effect
d. impedance effect

2 Which one of the following quantities varies the most with distance from the transducer face?
a. Axial resolution
b. Lateral resolution
c. Frequency
d. Wavelength

3 What determines the transducer frequency selection for diagnostic ultrasound?
a. Intensity and resolution
b. Intensity and propagation speed
c. Scattering and impedance
d. Resolution and penetration

4 Which of the following improves sound transmission from the transducer element into the tissue?
a. Matching layer
b. Doppler effect
c. Damping material
d. Coupling medium

5 The active elements of the diagnostic ultrasound transducer
a. may be crystalline material
b. operate on the basis of the photoelectric effect
c. convert electrical energy into mechanical energy
d. convert mechanical energy into electrical energy

6 The principle on which the ultrasound transducer operates is the
a. photoelectric effect
b. crystalline effect
c. piezoelectric effect
d. transducer effect

7 A piezoelectric crystal may be made of
a. aluminum
b. calcium tungstate
c. quartz
d. lithium fluoride

8 Best image resolution is obtained
a. at the transducer surface
b. in the near field
c. in the far field
d. in the focal zone

9 Crystals for ultrasound transducers are composed of
a. sodium iodide
b. quartz
c. barium titanate
d. lead zirconate titanate

10 The backing material in the transducer is
a. rubber
b. lead rubber
c. resin loaded with metal
d. plastic

11 The acoustic insulator in a transducer
a. is a safety device
b. reduces 'ringing'
c. is the main factor in shortening the pulse length
d. absorbs ultrasound

12 Phased array transducers
a. have elements which emit ultrasound independently
b. may be used to alter the beam direction

c. are used only on real-time scanners

d. have a variable frequency

13 A linear array transducer

a. has multiple elements of the same piezoelectrical material

b. can be used to produce real-time images

c. always has a frequency of 3.5 MHz

d. does not employ a coupling medium

14 Bandwidth

a. indicates the range of frequencies present

b. is related to the pulse length

c. is fixed for a particular transducer

d. is mainly determined by patient size

15 A coupling medium

a. is always used between the transducer and the patient's skin

b. is only used to help the transducer slide over the surface, thus reducing friction

c. eliminates air, thereby allowing maximum transmission of the beam

d. must be a water-soluble gel

Instrumentation

1 The dynamic range of an ultrasound system is defined as

a. the speed with which ultrasound examinations can be performed

b. the range over which the transducer can be manipulated

c. the ratio of the maximum to the minimum intensity that can be displayed

d. the range of pulser voltages applied to the transducer

2 The operation of the signal processor that reduces noise is

a. filtering

b. TGC

c. scan conversion

d. compression

3 Increasing the gain generally produces the same effect as

a. decreasing the attenuation

b. increasing the compression

c. decreasing output power

d. increasing the output power

4 The TGC control compensates for

a. focusing

b. machine instability

c. transducer aging

d. attenuation

5 Ultrasound is used in diagnosis to

a. produce dynamic images of physiological functions

b. demonstrate soft-tissue structures

c. monitor heart valve movement

d. produce three-dimensional images

6 Scan converters

a. are used only with conventional B scanners

b. may be either analog or digital

c. employ an electron gun and deflection system

d. increase the gray scale of the image

7 The dynamic range of an ultrasound system

a. is expressed in decibels

b. is a measure of resolution

c. expresses the range of the signal amplitudes that can be recorded

d. depends mainly on the frequency employed

8 Artifacts in B scanning can be caused by

a. reverberation

b. refraction

c. misregistration

d. room temperature changes

Doppler

1 The Doppler effect

a. measures the change in frequency of ultrasound

b. results from the movement of interfaces

c. may be used to determine blood vessel patency

d. is always detected in audible sound

2 The Doppler shift frequency

a. depends on acoustic impedance

b. is independent of the direction of movement of the interface

c. detected, will be greater at 5 MHz than at 2 MHz

d. is normally detected by a single transducer

3 The Doppler shift frequency is
  a. inversely proportional to the velocity of movement of an interface
  b. directly proportional to the pulse repetition frequency
  c. inversely proportional to the velocity of ultrasound in a medium
  d. dependent on the transmitted frequency

Safety

1 Ultrasound beams may produce
  a. cooling of the tissues
  b. cavitations
  c. cavitations independent of the frequency used
  d. streaming

2 Doses to the patient undergoing ultrasound examinations are increased
  a. if the pulse repetition frequency is increased
  b. if the intensity is reduced and the gain is increased
  c. when deeper organs are being visualized
  d. if the dynamic range is increased

3 In the exposure of the tissues to ultrasound
  a. the units of intensity are mW/cm^2
  b. the unit of ultrasound dose is the rad
  c. if the beam is said to have a 30 dB gain, that means it is 30% more intense than the reference beam
  d. if the reflected ultrasound beam is −40 dB, it is only 0.1% of the transmitted beam

MULTIPLE CHOICE ANSWERS

The Ultrasound Beam

1 An ultrasound beam passing through the body
   a. is attenuated
   b. produces heating of tissues
   c. can be reflected
   d. produces ionization

2 Ultrasonic pulses
   a. are poorly transmitted by liquids
   b. are poorly transmitted by air gaps
   c. are partially reflected at interfaces between two liquid media
   d. are partially transmitted at interfaces between two solid media

3 The Fraunhofer zone is the
   a. image plane
   b. image focus
   c. near field
   d. far field

4 Which of the following statements are true concerning the nature of diagnostic ultrasound in liver?
   a. The wave speed and frequency are constant regardless of the wavelength.
   b. The wave speed is constant regardless of the wavelength
   c. Wave speed increases with the increasing frequency
   d. None of the above

5 Which of the following characteristics of diagnostic ultrasound applies also to X-radiation?
   a. It is a wave phenomenon
   b. Its wave speed and frequency are inversely proportional
   c. Matter must be present for transmission
   d. Molecular compression and rarefaction occur

6 When two or more (plane) ultrasound waves exist in the same medium at the same time
   a. they will interfere constructively if traveling with the same direction and phase
   b. standing waves will be produced if they are traveling with the same direction and phase
   c. standing waves will be produced if they are traveling in the same direction but out of phase
   d. None of the above

7 Specific acoustic impedance as applied to diagnostic ultrasound increases with increasing
   a. frequency
   b. wavelength
   c. mass
   d. density

8 When the diagnostic ultrasound beam is incident on the surface separating different tissues
   a. none of the beam will be transmitted
   b. none of the beam will be reflected
   c. reflection can occur when the beam is at right angles to the interface
   d. when incident at greater than the critical angle, there will be total transmission

9 When an acoustic wave is transmitted through soft tissue
   a. there will be no reduction in intensity
   b. attenuation will occur
   c. energy will be transmitted by way of ionization and excitation
   d. energy will be transmitted by way of Compton scattering

10 When an ultrasound beam is attenuated while passing through tissue
   a. a 3 dB loss is equivalent to a 50% reduction in intensity
   b. a 6 dB loss is equivalent to a 100% reduction in intensity
   c. the normal rate is 10 dB/cm/MHz
   d. 90% reduction of the original intensity is equivalent to a 90 dB loss

11 When a transmitted ultrasound beam changes direction across an interface, this is called
   a. reflection
   b. defraction
   c. refraction
   d. scattering

12 Ultrasound and X-rays differ in which of the following ways?
  a. One is transverse, the other longitudinal
  b. One requires matter, the other does not
  c. One has constant wave speed, the other variable wave speed (in soft tissue)
  d. All of the above

13 Diagnostic ultrasound intensity is often measured in
  a. W/cm^2
  b. grays
  c. rad
  d. decibels

14 Intensity is equal to
  a. power/area
  b. area/power
  c. amplitude/distance
  d. frequency/wavelength

15 Diagnostic ultrasound intensity
  a. increases with increasing frequency
  b. is a measure of particle displacement in the conduction medium
  c. is measured in mW/cm^2
  d. is the same as ultrasound power

16 As ultrasound is transmitted through tissue, its intensity decreases because of
  a. excitation
  b. absorption
  c. scattering
  d. divergence

17 Acoustic reflectivity
  a. is determined by acoustic impedance at an interface
  b. equals 100 if $Z_1 = Z_2$
  c. is higher for an air–soft-tissue interface than a bone–soft-tissue interface
  d. increases with increasing frequency

18 An ultrasound wave may be described as
  a. a longitudinal pressure wave
  b. a transverse wave
  c. being formed by particle oscillations
  d. changes in electrical properties of tissues

19 Ultrasound used for diagnosis
  a. has a frequency in the region 2 to 10 kHz
  b. has a velocity in air of 1500 ms^{-1}

  c. will not travel through a vacuum
  d. is produced and detected by a transducer

20 Ultrasound has the following properties. It
  a. can be deflected by a magnetic field
  b. is attenuated in tissue
  c. has a sinusoidal wave form
  d. can travel through water

21 An ultrasound beam is attenuated
  a. by reflection at a tissue interface
  b. and causes ionization of atoms
  c. by scattering
  d. by absorption in tissues

22 Greater than 50% energy reflection will take place at a
  a. soft-tissue–bone interface
  b. water–soft-tissue interface
  c. soft-tissue–gas interface
  d. muscle–fat interface

23 The magnitude of the reflected signal
  a. decreases as the angle of incidence approaches 90 degrees
  b. depends on the change of acoustic impedance at an interface
  c. is independent of the acoustic impedance
  d. depends on the frequency of the beam

24 Interference phenomena
  a. may occur when two waves interact
  b. are more common with continuous wave ultrasound
  c. always produce a wave form of reduced amplitude
  d. may be of value to ultrasound

25 Acoustic impedance depends on
  a. the intensity of the ultrasound beam
  b. the elasticity of the tissue
  c. tissue density
  d. tissue temperature

26 In which of the following materials is the speed of ultrasound greatest?
  a. Air
  b. Bone
  c. Water
  d. Soft tissue

27 What is the wavelength of a 5 MHz ultrasound pulse in soft tissue?
   a. 0.3 mm
   b. 0.5 mm
   c. 3 mm
   d. 5 mm

28 As frequency increases
   a. wavelength increases
   b. imaging depth decreases
   c. propagation speed decreases
   d. a and b

29 The frequency of a sound wave is determined by
   a. the media through which it travels
   b. its propagation
   c. its source
   d. reflection

30 As frequency increases, the attenuation coefficient
   a. decreases
   b. increases
   c. stays the same
   d. attenuation coefficient not affected by frequency

31 Which of the following sound frequencies would include diagnostic ultrasound?
   a. 10 Hz
   b. 10 kHz
   c. 100 kHz
   d. 10 MHz

32 Velocity of ultrasound
   a. depends on the transmitted frequency
   b. varies for different materials
   c. is temperature dependent
   d. is equal for muscle and bone

33 The velocity of an ultrasound beam may be determined by measuring the
   a. time taken for a pulse to be returned through a Perspex block of a known thickness
   b. time taken for a pulse to be returned through a known depth of water
   c. reflection of the beam by a wire mesh placed in water
   d. distance between peaks of the wave form

34 The propagation speed of sound through soft tissue is
   a. 1450 ms^{-1}
   b. 1650 ms^{-1}
   c. 1540 ms^{-1}
   d. 1230 cms^{-1}

35 Given the various physical characteristics of ultrasound, then it is true that
   a. its speed is the same in all materials
   b. its speed does not depend on its frequency
   c. its speed depends on the density of the supporting medium
   d. its speed increases with frequency

36 Lateral resolution can be improved by
   a. damping
   b. pulsing
   c. focusing
   d. reflecting

37 Axial resolution can be improved by
   a. damping
   b. pulsing
   c. focusing
   d. increasing operating frequency

38 The resolution of an ultrasound beam may be determined by
   a. imaging a series of wires at varying depth from the transducer face
   b. imaging a series of wires all the same depth from the transducer face
   c. compound scanning around a Perspex block containing a single central wire
   d. linear scanning of a single wire in a water bath

39 The lateral resolution of the diagnostic ultrasound system is
   a. also called the azimuthal resolution
   b. determined by the slice thickness
   c. better with higher frequency
   d. better than axial resolution

40 The axial resolution of a transducer is primarily determined by
   a. spatial pulse length
   b. the transducer diameter
   c. the acoustic impedance of tissue
   d. density

41 The lateral resolution of a transducer is primarily determined by
a. spatial pulse length
b. the beam width
c. the acoustic impedance of tissue
d. applied voltage

The Transducer

1 The fundamental operating principle of medical ultrasound transducers is
a. Snell's law
b. ALARA principle
c. piezoelectric effect
d. impedance effect

2 Which one of the following quantities varies the most with distance from the transducer face?
a. Axial resolution
b. Lateral resolution
c. Frequency
d. Wavelength

3 What determines the transducer frequency selection for diagnostic ultrasound?
a. Intensity and resolution
b. Intensity and propagation speed
c. Scattering and impedance
d. Resolution and penetration

4 Which of the following improves sound transmission from the transducer element into the tissue?
a. Matching layer
b. Doppler effect
c. Damping material
d. Coupling medium

5 The active elements of the diagnostic ultrasound transducer
a. may be crystalline material
b. operate on the basis of the photoelectric effect
c. convert electrical energy into mechanical energy
d. convert mechanical energy into electrical energy

6 The principle on which the ultrasound transducer operates is the
a. photoelectric effect
b. crystalline effect
c. piezoelectric effect
d. transducer effect

7 A piezoelectric crystal may be made of
a. aluminum
b. calcium tungstate
c. quartz
d. lithium fluoride

8 Best image resolution is obtained
a. at the transducer surface
b. in the near field
c. in the far field
d. in the focal zone

9 Crystals for ultrasound transducers are composed of
a. sodium iodide
b. quartz
c. barium titanate
d. lead zirconate titanate

10 The backing material in the transducer is
a. rubber
b. lead rubber
c. resin loaded with metal
d. plastic

11 The acoustic insulator in a transducer
a. is a safety device
b. reduces 'ringing'
c. is the main factor in shortening the pulse length
d. absorbs ultrasound

12 Phased array transducers
a. have elements which emit ultrasound independently
b. may be used to alter the beam direction
c. are used only on real-time scanners
d. have a variable frequency

13 A linear array transducer
a. has multiple elements of the same piezoelectrical material
b. can be used to produce real-time images
c. always has a frequency of 3.5 MHz
d. does not employ a coupling medium

14 Bandwidth
a. indicates the range of frequencies present
b. is related to the pulse length
c. is fixed for a particular transducer
d. is mainly determined by patient size

15 A coupling medium
a. **is always used between the transducer and the patient's skin**
b. is only used to help the transducer slide over the surface, thus reducing friction
c. **eliminates air, thereby allowing maximum transmission of the beam**
d. must be a water-soluble gel

Instrumentation

1 The dynamic range of an ultrasound system is defined as
a. the speed with which ultrasound examinations can be performed
b. the range over which the transducer can be manipulated
c. **the ratio of the maximum to the minimum intensity that can be displayed**
d. the range of pulser voltages applied to the transducer

2 The operation of the signal processor that reduces noise is
a. **filtering**
b. TGC
c. scan conversion
d. compression

3 Increasing the gain generally produces the same effect as
a. **decreasing the attenuation**
b. increasing the compression
c. decreasing output power
d. **increasing the output power**

4 The TGC control compensates for
a. focusing
b. machine instability
c. transducer aging
d. **attenuation**

5 Ultrasound is used in diagnosis to
a. produce dynamic images of physiological functions
b. **demonstrate soft-tissue structures**
c. **monitor heart valve movement**
d. **produce three-dimensional images**

6 Scan converters
a. are used only with conventional B scanners
b. **may be either analog or digital**
c. **employ an electron gun and deflection system**
d. **increase the gray scale of the image**

7 The dynamic range of an ultrasound system
a. **is expressed in decibels**
b. is a measure of resolution
c. **expresses the range of the signal amplitudes that can be recorded**
d. depends mainly on the frequency employed

8 Artifacts in B scanning can be caused by
a. **reverberation**
b. **refraction**
c. **misregistration**
d. room temperature changes

Doppler

1 The Doppler effect
a. **measures the change in frequency of ultrasound**
b. **results from the movement of interfaces**
c. **may be used to determine blood vessel patency**
d. is always detected in audible sound

2 The Doppler shift frequency
a. depends on acoustic impedance
b. is independent of the direction of movement of the interface
c. **detected, will be greater at 5 MHz than at 2 MHz**
d. is normally detected by a single transducer

3 The Doppler shift frequency is
a. inversely proportional to the velocity of movement of an interface
b. directly proportional to the pulse repetition frequency
c. **inversely proportional to the velocity of ultrasound in a medium**
d. **dependent on the transmitted frequency**

Safety

1 Ultrasound beams may produce
a. cooling of the tissues
b. cavitations
c. cavitations independent of the frequency used
d. streaming

2 Doses to the patient undergoing ultrasound examinations are increased
a. if the pulse repetition frequency is increased
b. if the intensity is reduced and the gain is increased

c. when deeper organs are being visualized
d. if the dynamic range is increased

3 In the exposure of the tissues to ultrasound
a. the units of intensity are mW/cm^2
b. the unit of ultrasound dose is the rad
c. if the beam is said to have a 30 dB gain, that means it is 30% more intense than the reference beam
d. if the reflected ultrasound beam is −40 dB, it is only 0.1% of the transmitted beam

Index

Printed in the United States
By Bookmasters